T0259383

Quantitative Assessment of Musculoskeletal Conditions in Standard Clinical Care

Guest Editors

THEODORE PINCUS, MD
YUSUF YAZICI, MD

RHEUMATIC DISEASE CLINICS OF NORTH AMERICA

www.rheumatic.theclinics.com

Consulting Editor
ANTHONY WOOLF, BSc

November 2009 • Volume 35 • Number 4

SAUNDERS an imprint of ELSEVIER, Inc.

W.B. SAUNDERS COMPANY

A Division of Elsevier Inc.

1600 John F. Kennedy Blvd., Suite 1800 • Philadelphia, PA 19103-2899

http://www.theclinics.com

RHEUMATIC DISEASE CLINICS OF NORTH AMERICA Volume 35, Number 4

November 2009 ISSN 0889-857X, ISBN 13: 978-1-4377-0934-6, ISBN 10: 1-4377-0934-6

Editor: Rachel Glover

© 2009 Elsevier ■ All rights reserved.

This journal and the individual contributions contained in it are protected under copyright by Elsevier, and the following terms and conditions apply to their use:

Photocopying

Single photocopies of single articles may be made for personal use as allowed by national copyright laws. Permission of the Publisher and payment of a fee is required for all other photocopying, including multiple or systematic copying, copying for advertising or promotional purposes, resale, and all forms of document delivery. Special rates are available for educational institutions that wish to make photocopies for non-profit educational classroom use. For information on how to seek permission visit www.elsevier.com/permissions or call: (+44) 1865 843830 (UK)/ (+1) 215 239 3804 (USA).

Derivative Works

Subscribers may reproduce tables of contents or prepare lists of articles including abstracts for internal circulation within their institutions. Permission of the Publisher is required for resale or distribution outside the institution. Permission of the Publisher is required for all other derivative works, including compilations and translations (please consult www.elsevier.com/permissions).

Electronic Storage or Usage

Permission of the Publisher is required to store or use electronically any material contained in this journal, including any article or part of an article (please consult www.elsevier.com/permissions). Except as outlined above, no part of this publication may be reproduced, stored in a retrieval system or transmitted in any form or by any means, electronic, mechanical, photocopying, recording or otherwise, without prior written permission of the Publisher.

Notice

No responsibility is assumed by the Publisher for any injury and/or damage to persons or property as a matter of products liability, negligence or otherwise, or from any use or operation of any methods, products, instructions or ideas contained in the material herein. Because of rapid advances in the medical sciences, in particular, independent verification of diagnoses and drug dosages should be made.

Although all advertising material is expected to conform to ethical (medical) standards, inclusion in this publication does not constitute a guarantee or endorsement of the quality or value of such product or of the claims made of it by its manufacturer.

Rheumatic Disease Clinics of North America (ISSN 0889-857X) is published quarterly by Elsevier Inc., 360 Park Avenue South, New York, NY 10010-1710. Months of issue are February, May, August, and November. Business and editorial offices: 1600 John F. Kennedy Boulevard, Suite 1800, Philadelphia, PA 19103-2899. Customer Service offices: 11830 Westline Industrial Drive, St. Louis, MO 63146. Periodicals postage paid at New York, NY and additional mailing offices. Subscription prices are USD 244.00 per year for US individuals, USD 414.00 per year for US institutions, USD 122.00 per year for US students and residents, USD 288.00 per year for Canadian individuals, USD 512.00 per year for Canadian institutions, USD 342.00 per year for international individuals, USD 512.00 per year for international institutions, and USD 171.00 per year for Canadian and foreign students/residents. To receive student/resident rate, orders must be accompanied by name of affiliated institution, date of term, and the *signature* of program/residency coordinator on institution letterhead. Orders will be billed at individual rate until proof of status received. Foreign air speed delivery is included in all *Clinics* subscription prices. All prices are subject to change without notice. **POSTMASTER:** Send address changes to *Rheumatic Disease Clinics of North America,* Elsevier Journals Customer Service, 11830 Westline Industrial Drive, St. Louis, MO 63146. **Customer Service: 1-800-654-2452 (US and Canada). From outside of the US and Canada: 314-453-7041. Fax: 314-453-5170. For print support, e-mail: JournalsCustomerService-usa@elsevier.com. For online support, e-mail: JournalsOnlineSupport-usa@elsevier.com.**

Reprints. For copies of 100 or more of articles in this publication, please contact the Commercial Reprints Department, Elsevier Inc., 360 Park Avenue South, New York, New York, 10010-1710; Tel.: (+1) 212-633-3813, Fax: (+1) 212-462-1935, and E-mail: reprints@elsevier.com.

Rheumatic Disease Clinics of North America is covered in *MEDLINE/PubMed (Index Medicus), Current Contents/Clinical Medicine, Science Citation Index, ISI/BIOMED,* and *EMBASE/Excerpta Medica.*

Printed and bound by CPI Group (UK) Ltd, Croydon, CR0 4YY

Transferred to Digital Print 2012

Contributors

CONSULTING EDITOR

ANTHONY WOOLF, BSc
Duke of Cornwall Rheumatology Unit, Royal Cornwall Hospital, Truro, Cornwall, UK

GUEST EDITORS

THEODORE PINCUS, MD
Clinical Professor, Division of Rheumatology, Department of Medicine, New York
University School of Medicine and NYU Hospital for Joint Diseases, New York,
New York

YUSUF YAZICI, MD
Division of Rheumatology, Department of Medicine, New York University School
of Medicine and NYU Hospital for Joint Diseases, New York, New York

AUTHORS

DANIEL ALETAHA, MD, MS
Associate Professor, Division of Rheumatology, Department of Internal Medicine III,
Medical University of Vienna, Vienna, Austria

ANCA DINU ASKANASE, MD, MPH
Clinical Professor of Medicine, Division of Rheumatology, Department of Medicine,
New York University School of Medicine and NYU Hospital for Joint Diseases, New York,
New York

MARTIN J. BERGMAN, MD
Division of Rheumatology, Taylor Hospital, Ridley Park, Pennsylvania

LEIGH F. CALLAHAN, PhD
School of Medicine and School of Public Health, University of North Carolina
at Chapel Hill, Chapel Hill, North Carolina

JAAP FRANSEN, PhD
Department of Rheumatology, Radboud University Nijmegen Medical Centre, Nijmegen,
The Netherlands

AFTON L. HASSETT, PsyD
Division of Rheumatology and Connective Tissue Research, Department of Medicine,
UMDNJ-Robert Wood Johnson Medical School, New Brunswick, New Jersey

ROSS MacLEAN, MD
Bristol-Myers Squibb, Princeton, New Jersey

ARTHUR M. MANDELIN II, MD, PhD
Division of Rheumatology, Department of Medicine, Feinberg School of Medicine,
Northwestern University, Chicago, Illinois

LAUREN McCOLLUM, BA
Division of Rheumatology, Department of Medicine, New York University School
of Medicine and NYU Hospital for Joint Diseases, New York, New York

ALYCE M. OLIVER, MD, PhD
Section of Rheumatology, Department of Medicine, Medical College of Georgia, Augusta,
Georgia

THEODORE PINCUS, MD
Clinical Professor, Division of Rheumatology, Department of Medicine, New York
University School of Medicine, New York, New York; Division of Rheumatology, NYU
Hospital for Joint Diseases, New York, New York

JOSEF S. SMOLEN, MD
Chief, Division of Rheumatology, Department of Internal Medicine III, Medical University
of Vienna, Vienna, Austria

TUULIKKI SOKKA, MD, PhD
Jyväskylä Central Hospital, Jyväskylä, and Medcare Oy, Äänekoski, Finland

CHRISTOPHER J. SWEARINGEN, PhD
Department of Pediatrics, Biostatistics Program, University of Arkansas for Medical
Sciences, Little Rock, Arkansas

PIET L.C.M van RIEL, MD, PhD
Department of Rheumatology, Radboud University Nijmegen Medical Centre, Nijmegen,
The Netherlands

YUSUF YAZICI, MD
Division of Rheumatology, Department of Medicine, New York University School
of Medicine and NYU Hospital for Joint Diseases, New York, New York

Contents

The clinical approach to patients with inflammatory rheumatic diseases differs substantially from the approach to patients with many typical chronic diseases, such as hypertension or diabetes. Further elucidation of these differences may be informative in efforts to advance quantitative scientific patient assessment and management in rheumatic diseases, with improved patient outcomes.

Modern medical care is based largely on a paradigm known as a "biomedical model," in which a single "gold standard" high-technology test guides clinical care. Patients with hypertension, diabetes, osteoporosis, and many other conditions often are unaware of their status in the absence of data from "objective" tests. By contrast, in rheumatoid arthritis (RA) and most rheumatic diseases, patients generally are aware of symptoms, and information from patients often is as or more important to taking direct clinical decisions than laboratory tests, imaging studies, or even physical examination data. Physical function on a patient self-report questionnaire generally is as significant as, or more significant than laboratory, imaging, or physical examination data in predicting severe outcomes of RA, such as work disability, costs, and mortality. Patient questionnaires may be viewed as contributing to a complementary "biopsychosocial model" that can overcome limitations of the traditional "biomedical model" in RA and other chronic diseases. Further relevance of a "biopsychosocial model" in RA and other rheumatic diseases is seen in evidence that socioeconomic status, most easily assessed as formal education level, identifies favorable or unfavorable clinical status and prognosis at high levels of significance. Socioeconomic status may be regarded as a surrogate for the importance of patient actions, in addition to actions of health professionals, in the course and outcomes of rheumatic and other chronic diseases.

A joint examination is prerequisite to a diagnosis of rheumatoid arthritis (RA), and quantitative counts of swollen and tender joints are the most specific of the 7 RA Core Data Set measures for patient assessment. Therefore, joint counts are weighted of greater importance than the other 5 Core Data Set measures in American College of Rheumatology response criteria and all RA indices in which it is included. Nonetheless, several limitations to the joint count have been recognized: (1) poor reproducibility with a requirement to be performed by the same observer at each visit; (2) likelihood to improve with placebo treatment as much or more than the other 5 RA Core Data Set measures; (3) similar or lower relative efficiencies than global and patient measures to document differences between active and control treatments in clinical trials; (4) improvement over 5 years while joint damage and functional disability may progress; (5) lower sensitivity in detecting inflammatory activity than ultrasound and magnetic resonance imaging. Most visits to a rheumatologist do not include a formal quantitative joint count. Quantitative patient self-report data are as sensitive to change and as informative about prognosis and outcomes as joint counts. It may be suggested that a careful qualitative (nonquantitative) joint examination, supplemented by quantitative self-report questionnaire scores to interpret physical examination findings, may be adequate to monitor patients and document changes in status in busy clinical settings.

Yusuf Yazici, Tuulikki Sokka, and Theodore Pincus

Radiographs present several attractive features for the assessment and monitoring of patients with rheumatoid arthritis (RA). Radiographic erosions are the closest to a pathognomonic sign in RA. Radiographs provide a permanent record of permanent damage. Excellent quantitative scoring systems have been developed by Larsen, Sharp, van der Heijde, Genant, Rau, and others. However, quantitative radiographic scoring is used only in research studies and is not included in usual treatment. Furthermore, magnetic resonance imaging and ultrasonography may be more sensitive than radiography in detecting abnormalities. Moreover, treatment of patients with RA should be initiated before evidence of damage. Reports that biologic therapy is superior to methotrexate in preventing radiographic progression are accurate for groups of patients, although methotrexate and other disease-modifying antirheumatic drugs control inflammation in 70% to 80% of patients and most patients present no radiographic progression with methotrexate. Radiographic findings are also much less significant and functional measures are far more significant in the prediction of severe outcomes of RA, including costs and mortality. Whereas prevention of radiographic progression is certainly desirable, it appears that prevention of functional disability is far more important for successful patient outcomes.

Theodore Pincus and Tuulikki Sokka

Laboratory tests provide the most definitive information for diagnosing and managing many diseases, and most patients look to laboratory tests as the most important information from a medical visit. Most patients who have rheumatoid arthritis (RA) have a positive test for rheumatoid factor and anticyclic citrullinated peptide (anti-CCP) antibodies, as well as an elevated erythrocyte sedimentation rate (ESR) and C-reactive protein (CRP). More than 30% 40% of patients with RA, however, have negative tests for rheumatoid factor or anti-CCP antibodies or a normal ESR or CRP. More than 30% of patients with RA, however, have negative tests for rheumatoid factor or anti-CCP antibodies, and 40% have a normal ESR or CRP. These observations indicate that, although they can be helpful to monitor certain patients, laboratory measures cannot serve as a gold standard for diagnosis and management in all individual patients with RA or any rheumatic disease. Physicians and patients would benefit from an improved understanding of the limitations of laboratory tests in diagnosis and management of patients with RA.

In many chronic diseases, objective gold standard measures such as blood pressure, cholesterol, and bone densitometry often provide most of the information used to establish a diagnosis and guide therapy. By contrast, in inflammatory rheumatic diseases, information from a patient history usually is considerably more prominent in clinical management. Patient history data can be recorded as standardized, quantitative scientific data through use of validated self-reported questionnaires. Patient questionnaires address the primary concerns of patients and their families. Questionnaire scores distinguish active from control treatments in clinical trials at similar levels to swollen and tender joint counts or laboratory tests. Patient questionnaire data are correlated significantly with joint counts, radiographic scores, and laboratory tests, but usually are far more significant than these measures in the prognosis of severe outcomes of rheumatoid arthritis (RA), including work disability, costs, and premature death. Limitations of patient questionnaires are based on cultural features involving variation in responses among ethnic groups, and a need for translation, although translated questionnaires can be as valuable as a translator. Patient questionnaires do not replace further medical history, physical examination, laboratory tests, and imaging data, and they require interpretation in a context of these standard sources of information at any clinical encounter. Patient questionnaires are useful to monitor patient status in usual clinical care, with almost no effort on the part of the physician and staff if distributed by the receptionist in the infrastructure of office practice.

The Disease Activity Score (DAS), its modified version the DAS28, and the DAS-based European League Against Rheumatism (EULAR) response criteria are well-known measures of disease activity in rheumatoid arthritis (RA). The DAS is a clinical index of RA disease activity that combines information from swollen joints, tender joints, the acute phase response, and general health. The EULAR response criteria classify individual patients as non-, moderate, or good responders, depending on the extent of change and the level of disease activity reached. The DAS, DAS28, and EULAR response criteria have been validated extensively. For daily practice, it has been shown that a tight control strategy, including measurement of disease activity using the DAS and planned adjustment of

Indices of multiple measures have been developed to assess and monitor patients with rheumatic diseases, as no single "gold standard" measure is available for diagnosis, prognosis, and monitoring of all individual patients. Rheumatology indices generally include 4 types of measures from a standard medical evaluation: patient history, physical examination, laboratory tests, and imaging studies. Well-characterized indices are available for rheumatoid arthritis (RA), psoriatic arthritis, systemic lupus erythematosus (SLE), ankylosing spondylitis, vasculitis, osteoarthritis, fibromyalgia, and other rheumatic diseases. These indices are complex and applied widely in clinical research, but rarely are scored in usual rheumatology patient encounters, which generally are conducted without quantitative data other than laboratory tests. Information from a patient often is as prominent in clinical decisions as information from a physical examination or laboratory tests, and is easily collected as standardized "scientific" data on patient questionnaires designed for usual clinical care, which require minimal professional effort. Patient-derived data—along with physical examination, laboratory, and imaging data—are useful rheumatology "vital signs" to assess and monitor patient status, provide documentation, and improve the quality of clinical care, in addition to their possible value for clinical research. Differences between complex measures for research and simple questionnaires designed for usual clinical care might be more widely recognized, to promote quantitative measurement in the infrastructure of usual rheumatology care.

The health assessment questionnaire (HAQ) is the questionnaire most widely used to assess and monitor patients with rheumatic diseases. The HAQ includes 20 activities grouped into 8 categories of 2 or 3 (and queries the use of "aids and devices" and "help from another person" to perform these activities), and visual analog scales (VAS) for pain and patient global estimate of status. Use of the HAQ in usual care over the years has led to several modifications to develop a multidimensional HAQ (MDHAQ). The MDHAQ includes 10 activities, one from each category of the HAQ plus 2 complex activities—walk 2 miles or 3 km—all on one side of a page for easy "eyeball" review by a clinician; pain, global and fatigue VAS with 21 circles rather than 10-cm lines for ease of scoring; recent medical history; review of systems; a query about exercise; and scoring templates for the 3 rheumatoid arthritis (RA) Core Data Set patient-reported measures— physical function, pain, and global estimate—for a routine assessment of patient index data (RAPID3) composite score. Both the HAQ and MDHAQ involve 2 sides of one sheet of paper, and are completed by patients in 5 to 10 minutes. The HAQ requires 42 seconds to score, compared with 5 to 10 seconds for RAPID3 on the MDHAQ.

> Patient history data are prominent in rheumatology patient management and should be captured at each visit as standard, quantitative, scientific data by a self-report questionnaire. Patient questionnaire data on a multidimensional health assessment questionnaire (MDHAQ) provide scores for physical function, pain, global estimate of status, and routine assessment of patient index data (RAPID3), which may be regarded as rheumatology vital signs. Patient questionnaires designed for usual clinical care, such as the MDHAQ, save time and improve the quality and documentation of the visit for the patient and the physician.

> Little attention has been directed to quantitation of clinical impressions and estimates of physicians. This article describes a one-page worksheet for completion by the physician at each patient visit. It includes a physician global estimate and estimate of change in status and four quantitative estimates for the degree of inflammation, degree of organ damage, and degree of fibromyalgia or somatization. An estimate of prognosis is recorded, with no therapy and with available therapies. All changes in medications are recorded. A template is available for a formal 42 joint count. The worksheet requires fewer than 15 seconds and has proven of considerable value in clinical care.

> Although indices have been developed for many rheumatic diseases in usual care, they are rarely used in usual care. In most visits to rheumatologists, the only quantitative data collected are laboratory tests. Patient history data often are more important in management of patients with rheumatic diseases than other diseases. A two-page multidimensional health assessment questionnaire (MDHAQ) can be completed by the patient in 5 to 10 minutes and reviewed by the physician in 10 seconds, with RAPID3 scored in 5 to 10 seconds. The MDHAQ is useful in rheumatic diseases, to improve management documentation and outcomes. MDHAQ data for physical function, pain, global status, and RAPID3 scores appear preferable to no quantitative data.

> Electronic medical records (EMR) are used increasingly in contemporary medical care. Function, pain, global status, and RAPID3 scores remain

important considerations in all rheumatic diseases. Inclusion of these scores in a flowsheet that also includes laboratory tests and medications could transform the EMR into a true medical database. Flowsheets are presented for patients with rheumatologic diagnoses other than rheumatoid arthritis to illustrate the value of the multidimensional health assessment questionnaire and RAPID3 scores in an electronic database for an EMR.

An efficient, uniform procedure to collect essential data for patients who have rheumatoid arthritis (RA) using a two- to four-page patient questionnaire and a three-page form for health professionals is known as a *Standard Protocol to Assess Rheumatoid Arthritis* (SPERA). The two- to four-page patient questionnaire may be a health assessment questionnaire (HAQ), multidimensional HAQ (MDHAQ), or variant, including a four-page format used in the Questionnaire in Standard Care of Patients with Rheumatoid Arthritis (QUEST-RA) program. On each page, the three-page form for health professionals addresses (1) clinical features of RA; (2) medications taken currently, and major disease-modifying antirheumatic drugs (DMARDs) taken previously; and (3) a 42-joint count, with joints assessed for four variables: swelling, tenderness, deformity/limited motion, and surgeries, and an entry for no abnormality. A radiographic scoring sheet may be included for a comprehensive baseline database. The 15 to 20 minutes needed to complete the SPERA generally produces efficiency over time in standard clinical care and does not preclude collection of additional information for clinical research or clinical care. The SPERA is presented as an example of a possible approach to develop a uniform common format for collecting core data in usual clinical care.

A method is summarized to improve quality control of the patient history in the medical record, incorporating the patient as a partner to review and correct the information. This method has been implemented at every patient visit to the senior author since 2000, in the infrastructure of usual medical care, using a database. This procedure engenders a more accurate patient history with no effort on the part of the physician, saving time for the physician and improving the quality of the medical record.

The validity of information on a patient questionnaire may not necessarily be generalizable to all individuals and situations, and may depend on the context in which a person provides the information. Examples may be seen in responses of people with rheumatoid arthritis on the Minnesota Multiphasic Personality Inventory (MMPI), on the original Beck Depression Inventory (BDI), and on the Centers for Epidemiologic Studies Depression Scale (CES-D). Several reports have indicated tendencies toward hypochondriasis, depression, and/or hysteria on the MMPI, and tendencies toward depression on the original BDI and CES-D. However, these interpretations were based in large part on responses to such statements as "I am in just as good physical health as most of my friends," "I can work about as well as before," and "I could not get going." These responses would suggest psychological concerns in people who have no somatic disease, the type of subjects in whom these scales were validated, but would also appear appropriate for people with rheumatoid arthritis, including those with no psychological problems. Rheumatologists confirmed independently the likelihood that people with rheumatoid arthritis would respond differently from the general population in responding to these and other statements. This phenomenon, known as *criterion contamination*, would explain much, but not all, of elevations in scores on these scales in patients with rheumatoid arthritis. The BDI was revised in 1996, as the Beck Depression Inventory-II (BDI-II), to eliminate the items reflecting somatic disease.

Patients with fibromyalgia and chronic pain conditions report high levels of pain and fatigue, and multiple symptoms. These phenomena may be recorded quantitatively on a self-report multidimensional health assessment questionnaire (MDHAQ). These responses are likely to differ in people with fibromyalgia or chronic pain conditions compared with people with an inflammatory rheumatic disease, such as rheumatoid arthritis. Data from the MDHAQ provide clues to the presence of fibromyalgia/chronic pain conditions, including patients with inflammatory diseases who also have concomitant fibromyalgia/chronic pain conditions.

THE CLINICS ARE NOW AVAILABLE ONLINE!

Access your subscription at:
www.theclinics.com

Complexities in Assessment of Rheumatoid Arthritis: Absence of a Single Gold Standard Measure

Theodore Pincus, MD[a],*, Yusuf Yazici, MD[a],
Tuulikki Sokka, MD, PhD[b]

KEYWORDS

- Laboratory tests • Patient questionnaires
- Classification criteria • Assessment indices

The clinical approach to rheumatic diseases differs considerably from the approach to typical chronic diseases in several important respects (**Box 1**). Further recognition of these differences may be informative in efforts to advance quantitative scientific patient assessment and management in rheumatic diseases, leading to improved patient outcomes.

ABSENCE OF A GOLD STANDARD IN RHEUMATIC DISEASES

Quantitative assessment and monitoring of typical chronic diseases, such as hypertension, diabetes, and osteoporosis, is characterized by a gold standard measure, such as blood pressure, hemoglobin A_{1c}, and bone density, to provide the primary information for diagnosis, assessment, prognosis, and monitoring for clinical decisions. Tight control according to this gold standard measure has been documented to result in better patient outcomes, including improved survival, largely, in many diseases. A patient history and physical examination are limited and often irrelevant

A version of this article originally appeared in the 21:4 issue of *Best Practice & Research Clinical Rheumatology*.

Supported in part by grants from the Arthritis Foundation, the Jack C. Massey Foundation, Bristol-Myers Squibb, and Amgen.

[a] Division of Rheumatology, Department of Medicine, New York University School of Medicine and NYU Hospital for Joint Diseases, 301 East 17th Street, Room 1608, New York, NY 10003, USA

[b] Jyväskylä Central Hospital, Jyväskylä, and Medcare Oy, Äänekoski, Finland

* Corresponding author.

E-mail address: tedpincus@gmail.com (T. Pincus).

Rheum Dis Clin N Am 35 (2009) 687–697
doi:10.1016/j.rdc.2009.10.002
0889-857X/09/$ – see front matter © 2009 Elsevier Inc. All rights reserved.

rheumatic.theclinics.com

Box 1
Differences of rheumatic diseases from typical chronic diseases

1. Absence of a single gold standard measure, such as blood pressure, creatinine, and so forth.

2. Laboratory tests are neither as sensitive nor specific as gold standard measures, and normal in >30% of patients, including rheumatoid factor, anti–cyclic citrullinated peptide antibodies, erythrocyte sedimentation rate, and C-reactive protein in rheumatoid arthritis, and anti-DNA, anti-Smith, and antiribonucleoprotein antibodies in systemic lupus erythematosus.

3. Diagnosis, management, classification criteria, and indices for management incorporate four types of information from a patient history, physical examination, laboratory tests, and imaging studies, rather than a single primary measure.

4. Information from a patient history is considerably more prominent in management decisions in rheumatic diseases than in typical chronic diseases, for which patient history and symptoms often are irrelevant, and can be captured as standardized, quantitative, scientific data using a validated patient self-report questionnaire.

5. Definitive diagnosis is based on physician's judgment rather than an objective marker.

---

to management decisions, which are based largely, if not entirely, on the gold standard measure.

Rheumatologists have attempted to implement a similar approach to patients with inflammatory rheumatic diseases for more than half a century. The discovery in the 1940s of rheumatoid factor[1,2] in rheumatoid arthritis (RA), and antinuclear antibodies (ANA)[3] in systemic lupus erythematosus (SLE), led to hopes that laboratory tests could be used effectively for diagnosis and management of all individual patients with RA, SLE, and other rheumatic diseases. Indeed, laboratory tests are included in assessment of virtually every patient suspected of having an inflammatory rheumatic disease by both primary care physicians and rheumatologists. As of 2009, however, no laboratory test or any other quantitative measure can serve as a gold standard for all individual patients with any rheumatic disease.

SENSITIVITY AND SPECIFICITY OF LABORATORY TESTS IN INFLAMMATORY RHEUMATIC DISEASES

Laboratory tests are abnormal in most patients who have RA or SLE, and are helpful in many patients. More than one third of patients with RA have at presentation, however, a normal erythrocyte sedimentation rate, C-reactive protein, rheumatoid factor, and anti–cyclic citrullinated peptide antibodies (**Table 1**).[4–7] More than one third of patients with SLE have normal levels of anti-DNA antibodies, and ANA subset tests anti-Smith (anti-Sm) and antiribonucleoprotein (anti-RNP) (**Table 2, Fig. 1**).[8–10]

In addition to these false-negative results, ANA subsets indicate relatively little specificity for particular rheumatic diagnoses. For example, among a group of 150 patients with anti-Sm or anti-RNP antibodies, 64% of patients with anti-Sm and 51% of those with anti-RNP had a diagnosis of SLE (see **Table 2**). The percentages of patients with various other rheumatic and nonrheumatic diagnoses ranged from 1% to 12%, with little specificity (see **Table 2**).[8]

Information concerning autoantibodies and other biomarkers is invaluable in laboratory research to further characterize the pathogenesis, course, and outcomes of diseases, and to develop new therapies. Anti–tumor necrosis factor and other biologic

Table 1
Percentage of patients with rheumatoid arthritis who have abnormal laboratory tests

Test	Percentage of Rheumatoid Arthritis Patients with Abnormal Test Result (%)
Rheumatoid factor[a]	69
Anti-CCP antibodies[a]	67
ESR[b]	55
CRP[b]	56

Abbreviations: Anti-CCP, anticyclic citrullinated peptide; CRP, C-reactive protein; ESR, erythrocyte sedimentation rate.

[a] *Data from* Nishimura K, Sugiyama D, Kogata Y, et al. Meta-analysis: diagnostic accuracy of anticyclic citrullinated peptide antibody and rheumatoid factor for rheumatoid arthritis. Ann Intern Med 2007;146:797–08.

[b] *Data from* Sokka T, Pincus T. Erythrocyte sedimentation rate, C-reactive protein, or rheumatoid factor are normal at presentation in 35%–45% of patients with rheumatoid arthritis seen between 1980 and 2004: analyses from Finland and the United States. J Rheumatol 2009;36:1387–90.

agents emerged from efforts to characterize rheumatoid factor alpha (TNFa) and immunologic dysregulation in patients with RA. Furthermore, strong associations of clinical status with variation in biomarkers have been observed in some patients and reported by many rheumatologists, including the senior author. For example, treatment of a patient with SLE nephritis was reported in 1969 to result in a decline in anti-DNA antibodies and erythrocyte sedimentation rate, with a rise in serum

Table 2
Diagnoses in 150 patients with antibodies to Sm or RNP

Diagnosis	Anti-Sm: 42 Patients N (%)	Anti-RNP: 76 Patients N (%)	Anti-Sm and Anti-RNP: 32 Patients N (%)
Systemic lupus erythematosus	27 (64)	39 (51)	20 (63)
Cutaneous lupus	0 (0)	3 (4)	0 (0)
Drug-induced lupus	4 (10)	7 (9)	1 (3)
Rheumatoid arthritis	4 (10)	9 (12)	4 (13)
Juvenile arthritis	1 (2)	1 (1)	1 (3)
Mixed connective tissue disease	0 (0)	2 (3)	2 (6)
Raynaud disease	0 (0)	1 (1)	1 (3)
Progressive systemic sclerosis	0 (0)	1 (1)	1 (3)
Miscellaneous rheumatic disease	1 (2)	5 (7)	0 (0)
Undifferentiated connective tissue disease	4 (10)	4 (5)	0 (0)
Miscellaneous nonrheumatic disease	1 (2)	4 (5)	2 (6)

From Munves EF, Schur PH. Antibodies to Sm and RNP: prognosticators of disease involvement. Arthritis Rheum 1983;26:848–53; with permission.

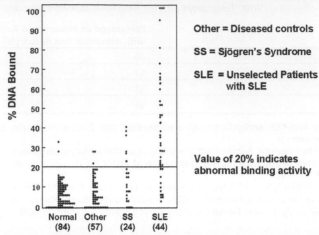

Fig. 1. Serum binding of DNA antibodies in patients with SLE, SS, or another diagnosis, and in healthy individuals. (*From* Pincus T, Schur PH, Rose JA, et al. Measurement of serum DNA-binding activity in systemic lupus erythematosus. N Engl J Med 1969;281:701–5; with permission.)

complement levels and creatinine clearance (**Fig. 2**).[11] This type of analysis is intellectually satisfying, apparently related to the pathogenesis of disease, and introducing the scientific method into standard rheumatology clinical care.

At the same time, rheumatologists, including the senior author, have conveniently ignored that laboratory biomarkers are not informative in all patients. For example, in the previously mentioned report concerning DNA antibodies,[11] although 50% of SLE patients and no control patient had binding to DNA greater than 50%, 25% of SLE patients were in the normal range of less than 20% binding (see **Fig. 1**). No biomarker is positive in 100% of patients with any rheumatic disease.

A further complexity in interpretation of laboratory test results in rheumatic diseases involves false-positive results, in which a test is abnormal in people who do not have a disease. Indeed, results of most tests that are regarded as important in the diagnosis of specific rheumatic diseases, such as rheumatoid factor, ANA, HLA B-27, and serum uric acid, are abnormal more frequently in the general population in individuals who do not have the associated disease than those who have this disease, sometimes 100-fold more likely in the case of an ANA.[9,10] Laboratory tests cannot provide a single gold standard measure for diagnosis, prognosis, monitoring, and outcomes assessment in every individual patient with a rheumatic disease.

DIAGNOSIS, CLASSIFICATION, AND MANAGEMENT OF RHEUMATIC DISEASES

In the absence of a single gold standard measure, the clinical approach to patients with inflammatory rheumatic diseases is guided by patterns of the four types of information used in standard clinical assessment: (1) patient history, (2) physical examination, (3) laboratory tests, and (4) imaging studies. These four types of measures are incorporated into formal classification criteria established to standardize patient enrollment in clinical trials and other clinical research studies for RA,[12] ankylosing spondylitis,[13] rheumatic fever,[14] osteoarthritis,[15,16] gout,[17] SLE,[18,19] systemic sclerosis,[20] polymyositis and dermatomyositis,[21] Sjögren syndrome,[22] vasculitis,[23]

Quantitative Monitoring of a Patient With SLE over 180 days: ESR, anti-DNA, CH50

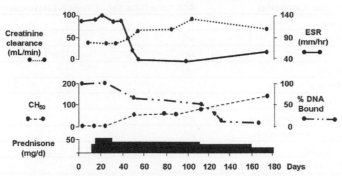

Fig. 2. Treatment of a patient with SLE nephritis results in a decline in anti-DNA antibodies, rise in serum complement levels, decline in the erythrocyte sedimentation rate (ESR), and rise in creatinine clearance. (*From* Pincus T, Schur PH, Rose JA, et al. Measurement of serum DNA-binding activity in systemic lupus erythematosus. N Engl J Med 1969;281:701–5; with permission.)

Behçet disease,[24] and antiphospholipid syndrome.[25] American College of Rheumatology (ACR) 1987 classification criteria for RA[12] include seven features (**Table 3**):

Morning stiffness
Arthritis of three or more joint areas
Arthritis of hand joints
Symmetric arthritis
Rheumatoid nodules
Serum rheumatoid factor
Radiographic changes

A patient is considered to have RA if four of these seven criteria are met over at least six weeks. New criteria were presented at the 2009 ACR meeting, and may have been published by the time this article is published.

The tetrad of patient symptoms, physical examination, laboratory tests, and imaging studies also is recognized in formal indices to describe clinical status in RA,[26–31] SLE,[32–39] vasculitis,[40–45] psoriatic arthritis,[46–48] ankylosing spondylitis,[49–53] and other rheumatic diseases. Indices for RA are based on a Core Data Set[54] of seven measures (**Table 4**): three from a physician (swollen joint count, tender joint count, physician global estimate of status); one laboratory test of an acute-phase reactant (erythrocyte sedimentation rate or C-reactive protein); and three from a patient self-report questionnaire (physical function, pain, and patient global estimate of status).

The most widely used index, the disease activity score 28 (DAS28),[26,27] includes measures from physical examination, laboratory, and patient self-report (see **Table 4**). The clinical disease activity index (CDAI)[28] (see **Table 4**) includes a physician global estimate in lieu of a laboratory test. Routine assessment of patient index data 3 (RAPID3)[30,31] (see **Table 4**) excludes both laboratory tests, on the basis of frequently normal values and unavailability, and a formal joint count, on the basis of many limitations[55] (see "Joint Counts to Assess Rheumatoid Arthritis" by Sokka T, Pincus T, in

Table 3
ACR Core Data Set[a] and ACR classification criteria for RA[b]

Measures in Four Categories	ACR Core Data Set	ACR Classification Criteria
Patient history		
Physical function	✔	
Pain	✔	
Global estimate	✔	
Morning stiffness		✔
Physical Examination		
Formal count of swollen joints	✔	
Formal count of tender joints	✔	
MD/assessor global	✔	
Arthritis of three or more joint areas		✔
Arthritis of hand joints		✔
Symmetric arthritis		✔
Rheumatoid nodules		✔
Laboratory tests		
Serum rheumatoid factor		✔
ESR or CRP	✔	
Imaging studies		
Radiograph	If more than 1 year	✔

A patient is considered to have RA if four of the seven classification criteria are met.

Abbreviations: ACR, American College of Rheumatology; CRP, C-reactive protein; ESR, erythrocyte sedimentation rate; RA, rheumatoid arthritis.

[a] *Data from* Felson DT, Anderson JJ, Boers M, et al. The American College of Rheumatology preliminary core set of disease activity measures for rheumatoid arthritis clinical trials. Arthritis Rheum 1993;36:729–40.

[b] *Data from* Arnett FC, Edworthy SM, Bloch DA, et al. The American Rheumatism Association 1987 revised criteria for the classification of rheumatoid arthritis. Arthritis Rheum 1988;31:315–24.

this issue) and nonperformance at most visits to a rheumatologist outside of research settings (see **Table 4**).[56] RAPID3 includes only the three patient self-report measures from the RA Core Data Set. Patient data usually are the most prominent information used in management decisions in RA, and can be scored in 5 to 10 seconds, compared with 108 seconds for a CDAI, and 114 seconds for a DAS28.[57] Other RA indices have been developed: the mean overall index for rheumatoid arthritis (MOI-RA),[58] which includes all seven Core Data Set measures; a simplified disease activity index (SDAI),[28] which includes the four CDAI measures plus a laboratory test; and the LUNDEX,[59] an index designed to incorporate patients' adherence to therapy.

PATIENT HISTORY IN MANAGEMENT DECISIONS IN RHEUMATIC DISEASES

In most diseases a patient history and symptoms are regarded as "subjective," "unscientific" information, the primary purpose of which generally is to identify an "objective" gold standard "scientific" measure, which provides the primary information to diagnose, assess, monitor, and guide clinical decisions. By contrast, in rheumatic diseases, information from a patient history is considerably more prominent in management decisions compared with typical chronic diseases.

Table 4
ACR Core Data Set measures and indices to assess and monitor patients with RA

ACR Core Data Set Measures	DAS28	CDAI	RAPID3
Physician/assessor measures			
1. 28 TJC	0.56 × sq rt (TJC28)	0–28	—
2. 28 SJC	0.28 × sq rt (SJC28)	0–28	—
3. Physician global estimate of status	—	0–10	—
Laboratory measures			
4. ESR[a]	0.70 × ln (ESR)	—	—
Patient self-report measures			
5. Physical function	—	—	0–10
6. Pain	—	—	0–10
7. Patient global estimate of status	0.014 × PTGL	0–10	0–10
Total	0–10	0–76	0–30

Abbreviations: ACR, American College of Rheumatology; ESR, erythrocyte sedimentation rate; RA, rheumatoid arthritis; SJC, swollen joint count; TJC, tender joint count.
[a] C-reactive protein may be substituted for ESR as laboratory measure.

A patient history can be captured as standardized, "scientific" quantitative data, according to validated self-report questionnaires (see "Patient Questionnaires Rheumatoid Arthritis" by Pincus and colleagues, in this issue). Patient questionnaires may be used effectively to guide management, document change in status, assess outcomes, and improve the quality of care, as discussed further in this issue (see "How to Collect an MDHAQ" by Pincus and colleagues; "Flowsheets that include MDHAQ" by Pincus and colleagues). Inclusion of a patient questionnaire at every visit of every patient may be used to record information that has a substantial impact on patient management as quantitative scientific data.

DIAGNOSIS BASED ON A PHYSICIAN'S JUDGMENT

A final important difference between rheumatic diseases and typical chronic diseases is that rheumatic disease diagnoses are based on the judgment of an individual physician, rather than a pathognomonic marker from a physical examination, laboratory test, biopsy, imaging study, or other measure, as is the case in most typical chronic diseases. For example, in compiling information concerning the prevalence of various autoantibodies in patients with RA, SLE, and other rheumatic diseases (see **Tables 1 and 2**; see **Fig. 1**), the closest thing to a "gold standard" an assignment is the designation of a diagnosis by a physician.

These differences in quantitative assessment of rheumatic diseases compared with typical chronic diseases underlie the complexity of diagnosis, management, prognosis, and documentation of outcomes, as discussed in greater detail in subsequent articles in this issue.

REFERENCES

1. Waaler E. On the occurrence of a factor in human serum activating the specific agglutination of sheep blood corpuscles. Acta Pathol Microbiol Scand 1940;17: 172–8.

2. Rose HM, Ragan C, Pearce E, et al. Differential agglutination of normal and sensitized sheep erythrocytes by sera of patients with rheumatoid arthritis. Proc Soc Exp Biol Med 1948;68:1–6.
3. Hargraves MM, Richmond H, Morton R. Presentation of two bone marrow elements: the "tart" cell and "L.E." cell. Proc Staff Meet Mayo Clin 1948;23:25–8.
4. Nishimura K, Sugiyama D, Kogata Y, et al. Meta-analysis: diagnostic accuracy of anti-cyclic citrullinated peptide antibody and rheumatoid factor for rheumatoid arthritis. Ann Intern Med 2007;146:797–808.
5. Wolfe F, Michaud K. The clinical and research significance of the erythrocyte sedimentation rate. J Rheumatol 1994;21:1227–37.
6. Keenan RT, Swearingen CJ, Yazici Y. Erythrocyte sedimentation rate and C-reactive protein levels are poorly correlated with clinical measures of disease activity in rheumatoid arthritis, systemic lupus erythematosus and osteoarthritis patients. Clin Exp Rheumatol 2008;26:814–9.
7. Sokka T, Pincus T. Erythrocyte sedimentation rate, C-reactive protein, or rheumatoid factor are normal at presentation in 35%–45% of patients with rheumatoid arthritis seen between 1980 and 2004: analyses from Finland and the United States. J Rheumatol 2009;36:1387–90.
8. Munves EF, Schur PH. Antibodies to Sm and RNP: prognosticators of disease involvement. Arthritis Rheum 1983;26:848–53.
9. Pincus T. A pragmatic approach to cost-effective use of laboratory tests and imaging procedures in patients with musculoskeletal symptoms. Prim Care 1993;20:795–814.
10. Pincus T. Laboratory tests in rheumatic disorders. In: Klippel JH, Dieppe PA, editors. Rheumatology. 2nd edition. London: Mosby International; 1997. p. 10.1–10.8.
11. Pincus T, Schur PH, Rose JA, et al. Measurement of serum DNA-binding activity in systemic lupus erythematosus. N Engl J Med 1969;281:701–5.
12. Arnett FC, Edworthy SM, Bloch DA, et al. The American Rheumatism Association 1987 revised criteria for the classification of rheumatoid arthritis. Arthritis Rheum 1988;31:315–24.
13. Dougados M, van der Linden S, Juhlin R, et al. The European Spondylarthropathy Study Group preliminary criteria for the classification of spondylarthropathy. Arthritis Rheum 1991;34:1218–27.
14. Special writing Group of the Committee on Rheumatic Fever Endocarditis, and Kawasaki Disease of the Council on Cardiovascular Disease in the Young, American Heart Association. Guidelines for the diagnosis of rheumatic fever: Jones criteria, updated 1992. JAMA 1992;268:2069–73.
15. Altman R, Alarcon G, Appelrouth D, et al. The American College of Rheumatology criteria for the classification and reporting of osteoarthritis of the hand. Arthritis Rheum 1990;33:1601–10.
16. Altman R, Alarcon G, Appelrouth D, et al. The American College of Rheumatology criteria for the classification of osteoarthritis of the hip. Arthritis Rheum 1991;34: 505–14.
17. Wallace SL, Robinson H, Masi AT, et al. Preliminary criteria for the classification of the acute arthritis of primary gout. Arthritis Rheum 1977;20:895–900.
18. Tan EM, Cohen AS, Fries JF, et al. The 1982 revised criteria for the classification of systematic lupus erythematosus. Arthritis Rheum 1982;25:1271–7.
19. Hochberg MC. Updating the American College of Rheumatology revised criteria for the classification of systemic lupus erythematosus. Arthritis Rheum 1997;40: 1725 [letter].

20. Masi AT, Rodnan GP, Medsger TA. Preliminary criteria for the classification of systemic sclerosis (scleroderma). Subcommittee for Scleroderma Criteria of the American Rheumatism Association Diagnostic and Therapeutic Criteria Committee. Arthritis Rheum 1980;23:581–90.
21. Bohan A, Peter JB. Polymyositis and dermatomyositis. N Engl J Med 1975;292: 403–7, 344–7.
22. Vitali C, Bombardieri S, Moutsopoulos HM, et al. Preliminary criteria for the classification of Sjogren's syndrome: results of a prospective concerted action supported by the European Community. Arthritis Rheum 1993;36:340–7.
23. Calabrese LH, Michel BA, Bloch DA, et al. The American College of Rheumatology 1990 criteria for the classification of hypersensitivity vasculitis. Arthritis Rheum 1990;33:1108–13.
24. International Study Group for Behçet's Disease. Criteria for diagnosis of Behçet's disease. Lancet 1990;335:1078–80.
25. Wilson WA, Gharavi AE, Koike T, et al. International consensus statement on preliminary classification criteria for definite antiphospholipid syndrome: report of an international workshop. Arthritis Rheum 1999;42:1309–11.
26. van der Heijde DMFM, van't Hof M, van Riel PLCM, et al. Development of a disease activity score based on judgment in clinical practice by rheumatologists. J Rheumatol. 1993;20:579–81.
27. Prevoo MLL, van't Hof MA, Kuper HH, et al. Modified disease activity scores that include twenty-eight-joint counts: development and validation in a prospective longitudinal study of patients with rheumatoid arthritis. Arthritis Rheum 1995;38: 44–8.
28. Aletaha D, Smolen J. The simplified disease activity index (SDAI) and the clinical disease activity index (CDAI): a review of their usefulness and validity in rheumatoid arthritis. Clin Exp Rheumatol 2005;23:S100–8.
29. Pincus T, Strand V, Koch G, et al. An index of the three core data set patient questionnaire measures distinguishes efficacy of active treatment from placebo as effectively as the American College of Rheumatology 20% response criteria (ACR20) or the disease activity score (DAS) in a rheumatoid arthritis clinical trial. Arthritis Rheum 2003;48:625–30.
30. Pincus T, Bergman MJ, Yazici Y, et al. An index of only patient-reported outcome measures, routine assessment of patient index data 3 (RAPID3), in two abatacept clinical trials: similar results to disease activity score (DAS28) and other RAPID indices that include physician-reported measures. Rheumatology (Oxford) 2008;47:345–9.
31. Pincus T, Swearingen CJ, Bergman M, et al. RAPID3 (routine assessment of patient index data 3), a rheumatoid arthritis index without formal joint counts for routine care: proposed severity categories compared to DAS and CDAI categories. J Rheumatol 2008;35:2136–47.
32. Petri M, Hellmann DB, Hochberg M. Validity and reliability of lupus activity measures in the routine clinic setting. J Rheumatol 1992;19:53–9.
33. Bencivelli W, Vitali C, Isenberg DA, et al. Disease activity in systemic lupus erythematosus: report of the Consensus Study Group of the European Workshop for Rheumatology Research. III. Development of a computerised clinical chart and its application to the comparison of different indices of disease activity. The European Consensus Study Group for Disease Activity in SLE. Clin Exp Rheumatol 1992;10:549–54.
34. Hawker G, Gabriel S, Bombardier C, et al. A reliability study of SLEDAI: a disease activity index for systemic lupus erythematosus. J Rheumatol 1993;20:657–60.

35. Hay EM, Bacon PA, Gordon C, et al. The BILAG index: a reliable and valid instrument for measuring clinical disease activity in systemic lupus erythematosus. Q J Med 1993;86:447–58.
36. Gladman DD, Urowitz MB, Goldsmith CH, et al. The reliability of the Systemic Lupus International Collaborating Clinics/American College of Rheumatology Damage Index in patients with systemic lupus erythematosus. Arthritis Rheum 1997;40:809–13.
37. Mosca M, Bencivelli W, Vitali C, et al. The validity of the ECLAM index for the retrospective evaluation of disease activity in systemic lupus erythematosus. Lupus 2000;9:445–50.
38. Swaak AJ, van den Brink HG, Smeenk RJ, et al. Systemic lupus erythematosus: disease outcome in patients with a disease duration of at least 10 years: second evaluation. Lupus 2001;10:51–8.
39. Lam GKW, Petri M. Assessment of systemic lupus erythematosus. Clin Exp Rheumatol 2005;23:S120–32.
40. Luqmani RA, Bacon PA, Moots RJ, et al. Birmingham Vasculitis Activity Score (BVAS) in systemic necrotizing vasculitis. Q J Med 1994;87:671–8.
41. Bacon PA, Moots RJ, Exley E, et al. VITAL assessment of vasculitis: workshop report. Clin Exp Rheumatol 1995;13:275–8.
42. Exley AR, Bacon PA, Luqmani RA, et al. Development and initial validation of the Vasculitis Damage Index for the standardized clinical assessment of damage in the systemic vasculitides. Arthritis Rheum 1997;40:371–80.
43. Whiting O'Keefe QE, Stone JH, Hellmann DB. Validity of a vasculitis activity index for systemic necrotizing vasculitis. Arthritis Rheum 1999;42:2365–71.
44. Stone JH, Hoffman GS, Merkel PA, et al. A disease-specific activity index for Wegener's granulomatosis: modification of the Birmingham Vasculitis Activity Score. Arthritis Rheum 2001;44:912–20.
45. Seo P, Min Y, Holbrook JT, et al. Damage caused by Wegener's granulomatosis and its treatment: prospective data from the Wegener's Granulomatosis Etanercept Trail (WGET). Arthritis Rheum 2005;52:2168–78.
46. Clegg DO, Reda DJ, Weisman MH, et al. Comparison of sulfasalazine and placebo in the treatment of ankylosing spondylitis: a Department of Veterans Affairs Cooperative Study. Arthritis Rheum 1996;39:2004–12.
47. Fleischer JAB, Feldman SR, Rapp SR, et al. Disease severity measures in a population of psoriasis patients: the symptoms of psoriasis correlate with self-administered psoriasis area severity index scores. J Invest Dermatol 1996;107: 26–9.
48. Kavanaugh A, Cassell S. The assessment of disease activity and outcomes in psoriatic arthritis. Clin Exp Rheumatol 2005;23:S142–7.
49. Dougados M, Gueguen A, Nakache JP, et al. Evaluation of a functional index and an articular index in ankylosing spondylitis. J Rheumatol 1988;15:302–7.
50. Calin A, Garrett S, Whitelock H, et al. A new approach to defining functional ability in ankylosing spondylitis: the development of the Bath Ankylosing Spondylitis Functional Index. J Rheumatol 1994;21:2281–5.
51. Calin A, Nakache JP, Gueguen A, et al. Defining disease activity in ankylosing spondylitis: is a combination of variables (Bath Ankylosing Spondylitis Disease Activity Index) an appropriate instrument? Rheumatology (Oxford) 1999;38:878–82.
52. Calin A, MacKay K, Santos H, et al. A new dimension to outcome: application of the Bath Ankylosing Spondylitis Radiology Index. J Rheumatol 1999;26:988–92.
53. Zochling J, Braun J. Assessment of ankylosing spondylitis. Clin Exp Rheumatol 2005;23:S133–41.

54. Felson DT, Anderson JJ, Boers M, et al. The American College of Rheumatology preliminary core set of disease activity measures for rheumatoid arthritis clinical trials. Arthritis Rheum 1993;36:729–40.
55. Pincus T. Limitations of a quantitative swollen and tender joint count to assess and monitor patients with rheumatoid arthritis. Bull NYU Hosp Jt Dis 2008;66: 216–23.
56. Pincus T, Segurado OG. Most visits of most patients with rheumatoid arthritis to most rheumatologists do not include a formal quantitative joint count. Ann Rheum Dis 2006;65:820–2.
57. Colglazier CL, Swearingen C, Kaell A, et al. Time to score indices to assess clinical status in RA: Disease Activity Score (DAS28), Clinical Disease Activity Index (CDAI), Easy Rheumatoid Arthritis Measure (ERAM) and Routine Assessment of Patient Index Data (RAPID3) in usual clinical care [abstract]. Arthritis Rheum 2008;58(Suppl):S750–1.
58. Makinen H, Kautiainen H, Hannonen P, et al. A new disease activity index for rheumatoid arthritis: Mean Overall Index for Rheumatoid Arthritis (MOI-RA). J Rheumatol 2008;35:1522–7.
59. Kristensen LE, Saxne T, Geborek P, et al. The LUNDEX, a new index of drug efficacy in clinical practice: results of a five-year observational study of treatment with infliximab and etanercept among rheumatoid arthritis patients in southern Sweden. Arthritis Rheum 2006;54:600–6.

A Biopsychosocial Model to Complement a Biomedical Model: Patient Questionnaire Data and Socioeconomic Status Usually Are More Significant than Laboratory Tests and Imaging Studies in Prognosis of Rheumatoid Arthritis

Lauren McCollum, BA, Theodore Pincus, MD*

KEYWORDS

- Self-report questionnaires • Biopsychosocial model
- Biomedical model • Prognosis

Modern medical care is based largely on a paradigm known as a "biomedical model."[1–4] In this model, the causes, diagnosis, prognosis, treatment, and outcomes of diseases are determined largely by physical or somatic variables (**Table 1**). Mind and body are distinct in the causation and outcomes of diseases. General health, the approach to disease, and outcomes are determined primarily, if not exclusively, by actions of health professionals and the medical care system, with relatively little contribution and responsibility on the part of individual patients.

A version of this article originally appeared in the 21:4 issue of *Best Practice & Research: Clinical Rheumatology*.

Division of Rheumatology, Department of Medicine, New York University School of Medicine and NYU Hospital for Joint Diseases, 301 East 17th Street, Room 1608, New York, NY 10003, USA

* Corresponding author.

E-mail address: tedpincus@gmail.com (T. Pincus).

Rheum Dis Clin N Am 35 (2009) 699–712
doi:10.1016/j.rdc.2009.10.003
0889-857X/09/$ – see front matter © 2009 Elsevier Inc. All rights reserved.

rheumatic.theclinics.com

Table 1
Comparison of "biomedical model" and "biopsychosocial model" of disease

	Biomedical Model	Biopsychosocial Model
Cause	Each disease has a single "cause"	Disease etiology is multifactorial: external pathogens, toxins, and internal host milieu, genes, behavior, social support
Diagnosis	Identified primarily through laboratory tests, radiographs, scans; information from patients of value primarily to suggest appropriate tests	A patient medical history provides 50%–90% of the information needed to make many, perhaps most, diagnoses
Prognosis	Also established most accurately based on information from high-technology sources, rather than from a patient	Information provided by a patient often is the most valuable data to establish a prognosis
Treatment	Involves only actions of health professionals, eg, medications, surgery	Must involve patient, family, social structure
Role of health professionals and patients in general health and disease outcomes	Health and disease outcomes are determined primarily by decisions and actions of health professionals	Health and outcomes of chronic diseases are determined as much by actions of individual patient as by health professionals

The biomedical model has been spectacularly successful in twentieth-century medical and surgical patient care. An excellent example is seen in antibiotic therapy for acute infectious diseases, in which a "cause" is identified through a microbiological culture, leading to rational treatment and a "cure," if the host is intact. Similar successes have been seen in pharmacologic treatment of hypertension, hyperlipidemia, gastroesophageal reflux, and many other diseases, as well as surgical advances in coronary bypass, joint replacement, and many other conditions.

A biomedical model also provides a primary foundation for the understanding of pathogenetic mechanisms in disease. Advances in therapeutics such as effective biologic therapies for patients with rheumatoid arthritis (RA) are based on a biomedical model. Further research according to a biomedical model will remain critical to future advances in prevention and treatment of diseases.

In a traditional biomedical model, a "gold standard" assessed by a health professional by a health professional, such as blood pressure, serum creatinine, bacterium, or biopsy, provides the essential marker for diagnosis, prognosis, and monitoring. Information from a patient history helps to identify which "objective" "gold standard" is needed to establish a diagnosis. After the results become available, patient history information often is regarded as largely irrelevant to treatment decisions.

In rheumatic diseases, many aspects of diagnosis and management reflect a biomedical model, and major advances in therapy have been developed according

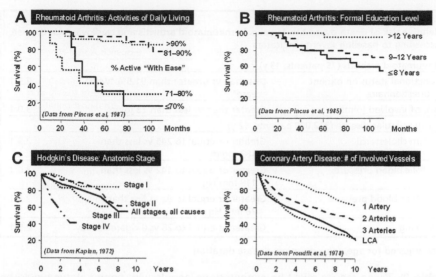

Fig. 1. Nine- to 10-year survival according to quantitative markers in 3 chronic diseases.[15,18,19]

to this model. However, certain aspects of rheumatic diseases reflect some limitations of a biomedical model. For example, no single gold standard is available for all individual patients. Furthermore, a patient history often provides important information for diagnosis, prognosis, monitoring, and outcome assessment. Patient history information may be recorded as standardized "scientific" quantitative data on validated self-report questionnaires (see "Patient Questionnaires in Rheumatoid Arthritis: Advantages and Limitations as a Quantitative, Standardized Scientific Medical History," by Pincus and colleagues, in this issue). Data from patient questionnaires are as effective as or more effective than laboratory tests and joint count data in discriminating active from control treatments in clinical trials.[5–8]

The most significant marker to predict premature mortality over 5 years in patients with RA is a score for functional capacity in activities of daily living on a patient questionnaire, rather than currently available laboratory tests, radiographs, or other imaging data.[9–17] In a study of patients who had an extensive baseline evaluation in 1973 and were reviewed 9 years later in 1982, patient responses regarding capacity to perform usual activities predicted mortality 5 years later more effectively than any known clinical measure (**Fig. 1**).[15] Patients who could perform fewer than 80% of activities of daily living "with ease" according to a questionnaire (**Fig. 1**A) experienced 5-year survival of about 50%, in the same range as patients with Stage IV Hodgkin's disease (**Fig. 1**C)[18] and 3-vessel coronary artery disease (**Fig. 1**D).[19] Patients with severe compared with mild RA, determined according to a questionnaire, have a 3:1 relative risk of death over the next 15 years (**Table 2**),[15] similar to the relative risk of death from cardiovascular disease according to the highest compared with the lowest quintile in the population for blood pressure, cholesterol, or smoking (see **Table 2**).[20]

A second cohort of patients was established in 1985 to attempt to determine whether patient questionnaires would predict mortality significantly if modern, quantitative measures of RA, including a 68-joint count, Sharp radiographic score, and laboratory studies were available.[21] All clinical measures indicated poorer status at baseline in patients who would not survive the 5-year period compared with survivors

Table 2
Relative risk of death over 12 to 15 years in rheumatoid arthritis and cardiovascular disease, according to baseline severity indicators

Rheumatoid arthritis (75 patients, 15 y)[15]		
Functional status on patient questionnaire	Less than vs greater than 91.5% "with ease"	2.9:1
No. of involved joints	Greater than vs less than 18 joints	3.0:1
Cardiovascular disease (312,000 patients, 12 y)[20]		
Serum cholesterol	Greater or equal to 245 vs less than 182 mg/dL	2.9:1
Systolic blood pressure	Greater or equal to 142 vs less than 118 mm Hg	3.0:1
Diastolic blood pressure	Greater or equal to 92 vs less than 76 mm Hg	2.9:1
Smoking	Greater or equal to 26 vs 0 cigarettes/day	2.9:1

Data adjusted for age, sex, education, disease duration.

(**Table 3**). These results might be expected, as people with poorer status would be more likely to die, although it may be regarded as an advance that poor versus good clinical status was expressed in *quantitative* rather than *qualitative*, descriptive terms (see **Table 3**).[21]

In this second cohort, the 3 independent predictors of mortality over 5 years in Cox regressions were age, comorbidities, and functional status according to a modified health assessment questionnaire (MHAQ) (**Table 4**).[21] All 12 patients who had normal scores of 0 survived 5 years, compared with 65% of 21 patients with scores of 2 or

Table 3
Predicting mortality in RA: most baseline measures are worse in patients who will die over a 5-year period[21]

Mean Baseline Values	Alive	Dead	*P* value
Age (y)	55.1	65.5	<.001
ARA functional class (1–4)	2.2	2.6	<.001
No. of comorbidities	1.1	2.1	<.001
Walking time (s)	10.8	16.8	<.001
ESR (mm/h)	33.8	48.3	.004
MHAQ score (0–3)[a]	0.98	1.32	.005
Learned helplessness (1–4)	2.41	2.55	.007
Global self-report (1–4)	2.6	3.0	.01
No. of extra-articular features	0.2	0.5	.02
Duration of disease (y)	9.1	12.7	.03
Years of education	10.8	9.4	.03
Joint count (0–66)	12.8	15.9	.04
Radiographic score (0–4)	1.2	1.4	.20
Log RF titer (0–12)	2.7	2.9	.28
Pain score (0–10)	5.40	5.19	.68

Abbreviations: ARA, American Rheumatism Association; ESR, erythrocyte sedimentation rate; MHAQ, modified health assessment questionnaire; RF, rheumatoid factor.
[a] Data changed from 1–4 in original report to 0–3 here reflects change in scoring since 1999.

Table 4
RA Cohort #2: 210 consecutive patients with RA in Nashville: Cox proportional hazards model analyses including demographic, functional, self-report, joint count, radiograph, laboratory, and disease variables[21]

	Univariate		Stepwise Model	
	Beta Coefficient	P	Beta Coefficient	P value
Age	0.072	<.001	0.061	<.001
Comorbidity	0.486	<.001	0.339	.018
MHAQ score	0.691	.002	0.566	.019
Disease duration	0.036	.02		
Education	−0.117	.007		
ESR	0.014	.005		
Joint count	0.023	.10		
Walking time	0.323	.04		
Radiograph	1.40	.17		

greater on a 0 to 3 scale (**Fig. 2**).[21] By contrast, minimal differences in 5-year survival were seen according to rheumatoid factor status (see **Fig. 2**).[21]

The observation that patient questionnaires predict mortality significantly, generally at higher levels than a joint count, radiographic score, or laboratory test, has been replicated extensively (**Fig. 3**).[11–14,16,17,21] Physical function was a significant marker for mortality in univariate or multivariate analyses in 94% (all but 1) of 18 studies in which it was included, and presence of comorbidities significant in 96% (also all but 1) of 23 studies in which it was included, compared with socioeconomic status in 77%, extra-articular disease in 73%, erythrocyte sedimentation rate (ESR) in 68%, rheumatoid factor in 66%, hand radiograph in 61%, and joint count in 50% of studies in which these variables were included. Patient questionnaire data also are as or more significant than joint counts, radiographs, and laboratory tests in predicting other severe long-term outcomes, including work disability,[22–24] costs,[25] and joint replacement surgery.[26]

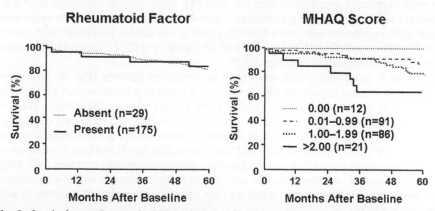

Fig. 2. Survival over 5 years in 206 patients with RA according to rheumatoid factor and functional status on a modified health assessment questionnaire (MHAQ). (*From* Callahan LF, Pincus T, Huston JW III, et al. Measures of activity and damage in rheumatoid arthritis: depiction of changes and prediction of mortality over five years. Arthritis Care Res 1997;10:381–94; with permission.)

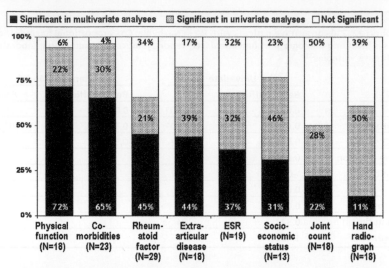

Fig. 3. Significance of 8 variables as predictors of mortality. In a review of 84 reports concerning mortality in RA, 53 cohorts presented predictors of mortality.[17] For each variable, n = the number of reports that included the variable, and bars indicate the percentage of those reports in which the variable was a significant predictor of mortality in multivariate analyses (*black*), in univariate analyses (*dotted*), or not significant (*white*).

A further challenge to a biomedical model involves evidence that the incidence, prevalence, morbidity, and mortality of RA and most chronic diseases are associated significantly with an individual's socioeconomic status, which may be assessed according to occupation, income, or formal educational level.[4] All 3 measures are correlated significantly, and associated with health; years of education is most easily assessed and generally the most significant socioeconomic variable.[27]

An association of formal education with mortality in RA was observed initially in the same cohort studied over 9 years from 1973 to 1982, in which physical function was the most significant predictor of mortality (see **Fig. 1**A).[19] Formal education level was a second significant predictor of mortality (see **Fig. 1**B).[19] Survival over 9 years was about 95% in patients with more than 12 years of education, compared with about 80% in patients with 9 to 12 years of formal education and 65% in patients with fewer than 8 years of education (see **Fig. 1**B).[28]

Declines in functional status were seen in almost all patients (**Fig. 4**), and were substantially greater in patients with fewer than 8 years of education than for patients with 9 to 12 years of education, which were in turn greater than those seen in patients with more than 12 years of formal education. Overall (**Fig. 5**), almost half of the patients with fewer than 8 years of education died over the study period, whereas fewer than 10% had the best outcome of less than a 20% functional loss, in contrast to patients with more than 12 years of education, among whom half had less than 20% functional loss and very few died. The association of poor outcome with low education level was accounted for only in small part by age, race, duration of disease, or any biomedical marker.[28]

Further evidence of associations between formal education levels and clinical status in patients with RA is seen according to all measures studied in a different cohort of 385 patients reported in 1988 (**Table 5**).[29] The mean ESR was 48 for individuals with 8 years or less of formal education, compared with 35 for high school graduates

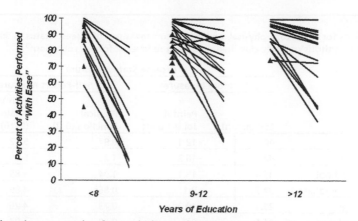

Fig. 4. Education as a marker for morbidity in rheumatoid arthritis. (*From* Pincus T, Callahan LF. Formal education as a marker for increased mortality and morbidity in rheumatoid arthritis. J Chronic Dis 1985;38:973–84; with permission.)

and 29.3 for individuals with some college education, although college graduates had a higher level of 42. The tender joint count (on a 0–28 scale) was 16.3, 15, 9, and 10 in the 4 education categories, respectively; physical function scores (on a 0–3 scale) were 1.26, 1.04, 0.86, and 0.73; and pain scores (on a 0–10 scale) were 5.75, 5.85, 4.89, and 4.26 (see **Table 5**). Patients with fewer than 11 years of education had at least a 2-fold higher likelihood of having poor clinical status than those with 12 or more years of education for all measures studied.[29]

Differences according to level of formal education were seen in scores for physical function and pain in patients with 5 different rheumatic diseases, RA, systemic lupus erythematosus, fibromyalgia, osteoarthritis, and scleroderma (**Table 6**).[30] Differences in both physical function and pain scores according to education level were greater than differences according to age or duration of disease (**Table 7**).[30] Nonetheless, almost every clinical report includes the patients' mean age and duration of disease, but fewer than 20% include a measure of patient socioeconomic status—20 years after this and other reports indicating similar findings![31–33]

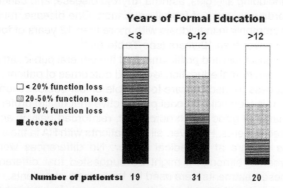

Fig. 5. Change in functional status over 9 years in rheumatoid arthritis. (*From* Pincus T, Callahan LF. Formal education as a marker for increased mortality and morbidity in rheumatoid arthritis. J Chronic Dis 1985;38:973–84; with permission.)

Table 5
Mean values for laboratory, physical, and self-report measures of disease status in 385
rheumatoid arthritis patients, classified according to level of formal education[28]

| | Disease Status Measure | | | |
| | Laboratory Measures | | Self-Report Measures | |
	ESR (mm/h)	Painful Joint Count	Physical Function (0–3)	Pain Visual Analog Scale (0–10)
All patients	40.1	12.1	0.97	5.12
Grade school	48.3	16.3	1.26	5.75
Some high school	49.4	15.1	1.04	5.85
High school graduate	34.7	9.1	0.86	4.89
Some college	29.3	10.2	0.73	4.26
College graduate	41.8	9.3	0.99	4.94
Postgraduate	26.6	8.5	0.70	3.86
P^a	.002[b]	.001[c]	.00[c]	.074

[a] By analysis of covariance, after controlling for age, sex, clinical setting, and disease duration.
[b] $P<.5$ after adjustment for multiple comparisons.
[c] $P<.1$ after adjustment for multiple comparisons.

In addition to associations of socioeconomic status with greater severity of disease and poorer outcomes after developing a disease, low formal education level is also associated with a considerably higher likelihood of *developing* most chronic diseases in Americans of age 18 to 65 years (**Table 8**).[34] For example, the 2 most common conditions in the United States population younger than 65, arthritis and hypertension, were found in about 25% of people with fewer than 8 years of education (about 10% of the 1978 total United States population younger than 65), 13% to 15% of people with 9 to 11 years of education (about 15% of the 1978 United States population), 9% to 11% of people with 12 years of education (about 38% of the 1978 United States population), and 6% to 7% of people with more than 12 years of formal education (about 37% of the 1978 United States population).[34]

Similar ratios were seen for most diseases, including back pain, heart attack, peptic ulcer, diabetes, chronic bronchitis, renal disease, epilepsy, stroke, and tuberculosis.[34] A few diseases, including allergies, asthma, thyroid disease, and cancer, did not vary significantly according to years of formal education. One disease, multiple sclerosis, was seen more commonly in individuals with more than 12 years of formal education than in those with fewer than 12 years (see **Table 8**).[34]

Most health professionals and politicians, and the general public, attempt to explain associations between formal education level and outcomes of patients with RA on the basis of limited access to medical care for people of low socioeconomic status. This explanation reflects a biomedical model perspective that health professionals are the primary determinants of good health outcomes, reinforced daily in acute-care situations in hospitalized patients. However, all the patients with RA in the studies reported here had access to care at a medical center. No differences were observed in prescribed treatments, although it might be suggested that differences may have existed in how these treatments were used by the individual patients.

It has been suggested that patient self-management, in contrast to professional medical intervention, may be the primary basis for associations between socioeconomic status and health.[27] Socioeconomic status may be a surrogate for actions of

Table 6

Responses of patients with five rheumatic diseases on two self-report questionnaire scales for physical function and pain, analyzed according to formal education level[30]

	Years of Formal Education	No. of Patients	Physical Function (0–3)	P value	Pain Visual Analog Scale (0–10)	P value
Rheumatoid arthritis	≤11	50	1.1	.005[a]	5.7	.12
	>12	83	0.8		4.9	
Osteoarthritis	≤11	82	0.7	.0002[b]	7.0	.001
	>12	124	0.5		5.5	
Fibromyalgia	≤11	23	0.9	.002[b]	8.1	.0004[b]
	>12	60	0.5		5.7	
Systemic lupus erythematosus	≤11	20	0.8	.0003[b]	5.9	.18
	>12	104	0.3		4.2	
Scleroderma	≤11	9	0.9	.04	5.5	.13
	>12	32	0.5		3.6	

[a] $P \leq .05$ adjusted for multiple comparisons using Bonferroni adjustment.
[b] $P \leq .01$ adjusted for multiple comparisons using Bonferroni adjustment.

Table 7
Regression analyses of responses of patients with 5 rheumatic diseases on 2 self-report questionnaire scales analyzed according to age, disease duration, and formal education level[30]

| | Physical Function | | | | | | Visual Analog Pain Scale | | | | | |
| | Years of Formal Education | | Duration of Disease | | Age | | Years of Formal Education | | Duration of Disease | | Age | |
	Beta	P	Beta	P	Beta	P	Beta	P	Beta	P	Beta	P
Rheumatoid arthritis	−0.17	.05	−0.06	.54	0.10	.30	−0.05	.54	−0.11	.24	−0.17	.07
Osteoarthritis	−0.16	.02	−0.02	.79	−0.01	.94	−0.22	<.01	−0.01	.90	−0.02	.79
Fibromyalgia	−0.33	<.01	−0.02	.88	0.10	.38	−0.18	.12	−0.06	.58	0.19	.09
Systemic lupus erythematosus	−0.37	<.01	0.00	.99	−0.01	.89	−0.16	.08	−0.07	.42	−0.12	.16
Scleroderma	−0.16	.32	0.06	.74	−0.20	.24	−0.21	.19	−0.03	.85	−0.05	.79

Table 8
Relative frequency of health conditions in the 18- to 64-year-old population according to level of formal education[34]

Health Condition	Total Number	% of Total Population	Percentage in 4 Categories by Years of Formal Education			
			1–8	9–11	12	>12
Any condition	54,194	42.7	64.7	53.5	41.3	33.4
Arthritis/rheumatism	14,215	11.3	26.4	13.1	11.0	6.8
Symmetric polyarthritis[a]	2,366	1.9	8.9	4.4	3.1	1.7
Asymmetric oligoarthritis[b]	4,261	3.4	14.2	9.7	7.0	4.3
Hypertension	14,015	11.1	26.1	15.1	9.5	7.2
Back problems	9,901	7.9	11.6	10.5	7.5	6.1
Nervous/emotional	7,203	5.8	16.8	9.4	5.4	1.6
Stomach ulcer	4,568	3.6	6.9	5.7	3.4	2.1
Diabetes	3,205	2.5	5.2	3.6	2.5	1.4
Kidney trouble	2,354	1.9	5.1	2.4	1.4	1.3
Chronic bronchitis	2,033	1.6	4.0	2.3	1.6	0.7
Heart attack	1,805	1.4	4.9	2.0	1.2	0.6
Cancer	837	0.7	1.5	0.6	0.6	0.5
Stroke	649	0.5	1.2	0.8	0.4	0.3
Multiple sclerosis	148	0.1	0.0	0.1	0.1	0.2

[a] Surrogate for rheumatoid arthritis.
[b] Surrogate for osteoarthritis.

a patient, which may be as important in health outcomes as actions of a health professional. Disparities in health according to socioeconomic status appear to be widening, rather than narrowing, over the last few decades in the United Kingdom,[35] the Netherlands,[36] and the United States.[37,38] Unequal access to medical care may explain differences in the United States and the Netherlands in small part. However, in the United Kingdom all citizens have access to a common medical system, the National Health Service.

Increases in health disparities according to socioeconomic status present a serious concern for modern societies throughout the world. It may be desirable that different treatment strategies beyond the routine encounter be developed for certain patients. The findings also suggest that rheumatologists should collect data concerning functional status using a patient questionnaire as a component of the infrastructure of routine care.[39,40] These approaches may require that the traditional biomedical model paradigm be broadened to recognize a biopsychosocial model of disease.

REFERENCES

1. Engel GL. The need for a new medical model: a challenge for biomedicine. Science 1977;196:129–36.
2. Pincus T, Callahan LF. Remodeling the pyramid or remodeling the paradigms concerning rheumatoid arthritis—lessons from Hodgkin's disease and coronary artery disease. J Rheumatol 1990;17:1582–5.
3. Pincus T. Challenges to the biomedical model: are actions of patients almost always as important as actions of health professionals in long-term outcomes of chronic diseases? [editorial]. Adv Mind Body Med 2000;16:287–94.
4. Pincus T. Patient questionnaires and formal education as more significant prognostic markers than radiographs or laboratory tests for rheumatoid arthritis mortality—limitations of a biomedical model to predict long-term outcomes. Bull NYU Hosp Jt Dis 2007;65(Suppl 1):S29–36.
5. Strand V, Cohen S, Crawford B, et al. Patient-reported outcomes better discriminate active treatment from placebo in randomized controlled trials in rheumatoid arthritis. Rheumatology 2004;43:640–7.
6. Cohen SB, Strand V, Aguilar D, et al. Patient- versus physician-reported outcomes in rheumatoid arthritis patients treated with recombinant interleukin-1 receptor antagonist (anakinra) therapy. Rheumatology 2004;43:704–11.
7. Pincus T, Amara I, Segurado OG, et al. Relative efficiencies of physician/assessor global estimates and patient questionnaire measures are similar to or greater than joint counts to distinguish adalimumab from control treatments in rheumatoid arthritis clinical trials. J Rheumatol 2008;35:201–5.
8. Wells G, Li T, Maxwell L, et al. Responsiveness of patient reported outcomes including fatigue, sleep quality, activity limitation, and quality of life following treatment with abatacept for rheumatoid arthritis. Ann Rheum Dis 2008;67:260–5.
9. Pincus T, Callahan LF, Sale WG, et al. Severe functional declines, work disability, and increased mortality in seventy-five rheumatoid arthritis patients studied over nine years. Arthritis Rheum 1984;27:864–72.
10. Söderlin MK, Nieminen P, Hakala M. Functional status predicts mortality in a community based rheumatoid arthritis population. J Rheumatol 1998;25:1895–9.
11. Sokka T, Hakkinen A, Krishnan E, et al. Similar prediction of mortality by the health assessment questionnaire in patients with rheumatoid arthritis and the general population. Ann Rheum Dis 2004;63:494–7.

12. Mitchell DM, Spitz PW, Young DY, et al. Survival, prognosis, and causes of death in rheumatoid arthritis. Arthritis Rheum 1986;29:706–14.
13. Wolfe F, Mitchell DM, Sibley JT, et al. The mortality of rheumatoid arthritis. Arthritis Rheum 1994;37:481–94.
14. Wolfe F, Michaud K, Gefeller O, et al. Predicting mortality in patients with rheumatoid arthritis. Arthritis Rheum 2003;48:1530–42.
15. Pincus T, Brooks RH, Callahan LF. Prediction of long-term mortality in patients with rheumatoid arthritis according to simple questionnaire and joint count measures. Ann Intern Med 1994;120:26–34.
16. Leigh JP, Fries JF. Mortality predictors among 263 patients with rheumatoid arthritis. J Rheumatol 1991;18:1307–12.
17. Sokka T, Abelson B, Pincus T. Mortality in rheumatoid arthritis: 2008 update. Clin Exp Rheumatol 2008;26:S35–61.
18. Kaplan HS. Survival as related to treatment. In: Kaplan HS, editor. Hodgkin's disease. Cambridge (Massachusetts): Harvard University Press; 1972. p. 360–88.
19. Proudfit WL, Bruschke AVG, Sones FM Jr. Natural history of obstructive coronary artery disease: ten-year study of 601 nonsurgical cases. Prog Cardiovasc Dis 1978;21:53–78.
20. Neaton JD, Wentworth D. Serum cholesterol, blood pressure, cigarette smoking, and death from coronary heart disease. Overall findings and differences by age for 316099 white men. Arch Intern Med 1992;152:56–64.
21. Callahan LF, Pincus T, Huston JW III, et al. Measures of activity and damage in rheumatoid arthritis: depiction of changes and prediction of mortality over five years. Arthritis Care Res 1997;10:381–94.
22. Callahan LF, Bloch DA, Pincus T. Identification of work disability in rheumatoid arthritis: physical, radiographic and laboratory variables do not add explanatory power to demographic and functional variables. J Clin Epidemiol 1992;45:127–38.
23. Wolfe F, Hawley DJ. The longterm outcomes of rheumatoid arthritis: work disability: a prospective 18 year study of 823 patients. J Rheumatol 1998;25:2108–17.
24. Sokka T, Kautiainen H, Möttönen T, et al. Work disability in rheumatoid arthritis 10 years after the diagnosis. J Rheumatol 1999;26:1681–5.
25. Lubeck DP, Spitz PW, Fries JF, et al. A multicenter study of annual health service utilization and costs in rheumatoid arthritis. Arthritis Rheum 1986;29:488–93.
26. Wolfe F, Zwillich SH. The long-term outcomes of rheumatoid arthritis: a 23-year prospective, longitudinal study of total joint replacement and its predictors in 1,600 patients with rheumatoid arthritis. Arthritis Rheum 1998;41:1072–82.
27. Pincus T, Esther R, DeWalt DA, et al. Social conditions and self-management are more powerful determinants of health than access to care. Ann Intern Med 1998;129:406–11.
28. Pincus T, Callahan LF. Formal education as a marker for increased mortality and morbidity in rheumatoid arthritis. J Chronic Dis 1985;38:973–84.
29. Callahan LF, Pincus T. Formal education level as a significant marker of clinical status in rheumatoid arthritis. Arthritis Rheum 1988;31:1346–57.
30. Callahan LF, Smith WJ, Pincus T. Self-report questionnaires in five rheumatic diseases: Comparisons of health status constructs and associations with formal education level. Arthritis Care Res 1989;2:122–31.
31. Ruberman W, Weinblatt E, Goldberg JD, et al. Psychosocial influences on mortality after myocardial infarction. N Engl J Med 1984;311:552–9.

32. Marmot M. Socioeconomic determinants of CHD mortality. Int J Epidemiol 1989; 18(Suppl 1):S196–202.
33. Pincus T, Callahan LF. Associations of low formal education level and poor health status: behavioral, in addition to demographic and medical, explanations? J Clin Epidemiol 1994;47:355–61.
34. Pincus T, Callahan LF, Burkhauser RV. Most chronic diseases are reported more frequently by individuals with fewer than 12 years of formal education in the age 18–64 United States population. J Chronic Dis 1987;40:865–74.
35. Marmot MG, McDowall ME. Mortality decline and widening social inequalities. Lancet 1986;2:274–6.
36. Kunst AE, Looman CWN, Mackenbach JP. Socio-economic mortality differences in the Netherlands in 1950–1984: a regional study of cause-specific mortality. Soc Sci Med 1990;31:141–52.
37. Feldman JJ, Makuc DM, Kleinman JC, et al. National trends in educational differentials in mortality. Am J Epidemiol 1989;129:919–33.
38. Pappas G, Queen S, Hadden W, et al. The increasing disparity in mortality between socioeconomic groups in the United States, 1960 and 1986. N Engl J Med 1993;329:103–9.
39. Pincus T, Wolfe F. An infrastructure of patient questionnaires at each rheumatology visit: Improving efficiency and documenting care. J Rheumatol 2000;27: 2727–30.
40. Pincus T, Yazici Y, Bergman M. Development of a multi-dimensional health assessment questionnaire (MDHAQ) for the infrastructure of standard clinical care. Clin Exp Rheumatol 2005;23:S19–28.

Joint Counts to Assess Rheumatoid Arthritis for Clinical Research and Usual Clinical Care: Advantages and Limitations

Tuulikki Sokka, MD, PhD[a], Theodore Pincus, MD[b],*

KEYWORDS

- Joint examination • Self-report questionnaire
- Joint count • Quantitative assessment

A careful joint examination is required to establish a diagnosis of rheumatoid arthritis (RA),[1] and quantitative counts of swollen and tender joints are the most specific measures for patient assessment.[2–5] The number of swollen and tender joints is regarded as the most important measure for RA clinical trials to distinguish active from control treatments,[6] and the best measure of status in usual clinical care.[7]

It might be ideal if a swollen joint count could serve as the *only* measure—a "gold standard"—to assess and monitor all individual patients with RA. However, some individual patients may have many swollen joints but little pain, whereas other patients may have considerable pain and few swollen joints, yet both may receive identical treatments. Therefore, the joint count is included in a Core Data Set[8–10] for pooled indices to assess individual patients (see "Complexities in Assessment of Rheumatoid Arthritis: Absence of a Single Gold Standard Measure," by Pincus and colleagues, in this issue).[11]

A version of this article originally appeared in the 21:4 issue of *Best Practice & Research: Clinical Rheumatology*.

Supported in part by the Arthritis Foundation, the Jack C. Massey Foundation, and Health Report Services Inc, and EVO-grants from Rheumatism Foundation Hospital, Heinola, Finland.

[a] Jyväskylä Central Hospital, Jyväskylä, and Medcare Oy, Äänekoski, Finland
[b] New York University School of Medicine and NYU Hospital for Joint Diseases, 301 East 17th Street, Room 1608, New York, NY 10003, USA
* Corresponding author. New York University School of Medicine and NYU Hospital for Joint Diseases, 301 East 17th Street, Room 1608, New York, NY 10003.
E-mail address: tedpincus@gmail.com (T. Pincus).

The primary indices that include a joint count, the disease activity score (DAS),[12,13] and clinical disease activity index (CDAI),[14] weight joint count data at higher levels than the other 5 Core Data Set measures. Nonetheless, several limitations of the joint count have been described, as with all quantitative measures (**Table 1**),[15–27] as summarized in this article and described in greater detail elsewhere.[28,29]

JOINT COUNTS ARE POORLY REPRODUCIBLE

Joint counts are poorly reproducible in formal studies.[15–27] For example, in one study interclass correlation coefficients for tender and swollen joint counts were found to be lower than seen for patient self-report questionnaire and radiographic scores (**Table 2**).[27] Similar results were seen in several other studies.[27]

Variation in joint count results can be reduced by training rheumatologists and other assessors to standardize scores.[21,25,26] Nonetheless, all protocols for clinical trials and other clinical research studies in RA require that a joint count must be performed by the same observer at each assessment. Most measures such as temperature, pulse, or blood pressure are regarded as ascertainable by any trained health professional at any time.

The need for the same person to perform each joint count in a given patient presents a serious limitation to use of joint counts as rigorous indicators of a need for changes in therapy, responses to therapy, or to document quality of care. Possible collaborative care between rheumatologists and family practitioners or other health professionals to manage patients is limited by a requirement for the same observer. By contrast, a patient self-report questionnaire always involves the same single observer—the patient.

JOINT COUNT MEASURES ARE AT LEAST AS LIKELY, OR MORE LIKELY TO IMPROVE WITH PLACEBO TREATMENT THAN THE OTHER 5 RA CORE DATA SET MEASURES

In clinical trials, patients who receive placebo or control treatments almost always show improvement according to swollen and tender joint counts as great as or greater than according to other Core Data Set measures.[30] For example, the last RA clinical trial conducted with a placebo (without "background" methotrexate or other disease-modifying antirheumatic drug treatment) compared leflunomide or methotrexate with placebo.[31] Placebo treatment resulted in improvement in patient status of 21% for swollen joint count, and 20% for tender joint count, compared wtih 12%

Table 1
Some limitations of joint counts

1. Joint counts are poorly reproducible,[15–27] with a need for the same observer to perform a joint count at each subsequent visit, excluding other health professionals

2. Joint count measures are at least as likely or more likely to improve with placebo treatment than the other 5 RA Core Data Set measures[30]

3. Joint counts have similar or lower relative efficiencies than global and patient measures to document differences between active and control treatments in clinical trials[30–40]

4. Joint counts may improve over 5 years while progressive joint damage and functional disability may occur[41]

5. Joint counts are not as sensitive in detecting inflammatory activity as ultrasound[59,61,62]

6. Most visits to a rheumatologist include a careful joint examination, but do not include a formal joint count[60]

Table 2
Reliability/reproducibility of joint examinations (interobserver reliability) and patient self-report clinical measures (test-retest reliability)[27]

Measure	Scale	Mean	ICC	Mean Difference
Joint examinations				
Tender 28	0–28	5.3	0.64	0.9
Tender 74	0–74	10.4	0.81	2.3
Swollen 28	0–28	5.1	0.52	1.0
Swollen 68	0–68	6.7	0.52	0.6
Patient self-report measures				
HAQ physical function	0–3	1.2	0.91	−0.05
Pain	0–100	37	0.75	−4.8
Patient global	0–100	37	0.75	−4.8

Abbreviations: ICC, interclass correlation coefficient; HAQ, health assessment questionnaire.

for physician global estimate of status and 12% for patient global estimate of status while worsening of status of 20% was seen for pain, 9% for physical function, and 22% for erythrocyte sedimentation rate (ESR) (**Fig. 1**). These data are typical of analyses of other clinical trials, which indicate that swollen and tender joint counts improve with placebo or control treatments as much as or more than other Core Data Set measures.

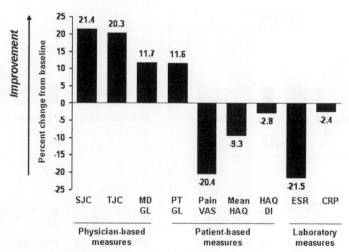

Fig. 1. Mean of the individual percentage changes from baseline in patient- and physician-reported measures for placebo patients at 6 months. The *arrow* to the left denotes improvement, indicating that deterioration in pain, physical function, and laboratory assessments were reported with placebo treatment. C-reactive protein (CRP) data exclude one outlier subject in the placebo group (percentage change more than 2 SD from the mean). ESR, erythrocyte sedimentation rate; HAQ, health assessment questionnaire; HAQ DI, HAQ disability index; MDGL, physician global estimate of status; PTGL, patient global estimate of status; SJC, swollen joint count; TJC, tender joint count; VAS, visual analog scale. (*Reproduced from* Strand V, Cohen S, Crawford B, et al. Patient-reported outcomes better discriminate active treatment from placebo in randomized controlled trials in rheumatoid arthritis. Rheumatology 2004;43:640–7; with permission.)

JOINT COUNTS HAVE SIMILAR OR LOWER RELATIVE EFFICIENCIES THAN GLOBAL AND PATIENT MEASURES IN DOCUMENTING DIFFERENCES BETWEEN ACTIVE AND CONTROL TREATMENTS IN CLINICAL TRIALS

Joint counts have similar or lower relative efficiencies in distinguishing patients who receive active versus placebo/control treatments in clinical trials, compared with other Core Data Set measures,[30–40] a consequence of apparent improvement of patient status associated with control or placebo treatments. For example, relative efficiency to distinguish active from control treatment was analyzed in 4 adalimumab clinical trials,[36] with arithmetic and percentage changes, resulting in 8 comparisons (**Fig. 2**). Efficiency relative to a tender joint count was greater for a physician/assessor global estimate in 8 of 8 comparisons, patient global estimate in 4 of 8, C-reactive protein (CRP) in 4 of 8, physical function in 3 of 8, pain in 3 of 8, and swollen joint count in 2 of 8 comparisons, while tender joint count was less efficient than other measures in all 8 comparisons. All Core Data Set measures have similar relative efficiencies to distinguish active from control treatments in clinical trials.

JOINT COUNTS MAY IMPROVE OVER 5 YEARS WHILE JOINT DAMAGE AND FUNCTIONAL DISABILITY MAY PROGRESS

Over 5 to 15 years, the numbers of affected joints may be reduced, but joint damage and functional declines may progress, leading to work disability and premature death.[41–51] In one study, 28 swollen and tender joint counts were improved over 5 years while joint deformity, limited motion, and radiographic scores indicated progression of damage

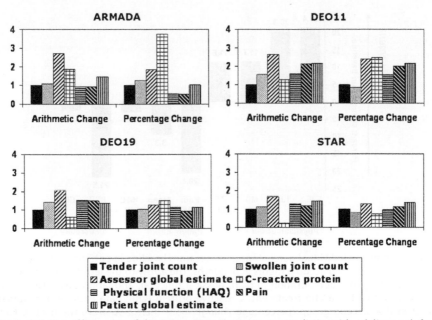

Fig. 2. Relative efficiencies of the 7 Core Data Set measures to distinguish adalimumab from control treatment in 4 clinical trials according to arithmetical and percentage changes. (*Reproduced from* Pincus T, Amara I, Segurado OG, et al. Relative efficiencies of physician/ assessor global estimates and patient questionnaire measures are similar to or greater than joint counts to distinguish adalimumab from control treatments in rheumatoid arthritis clinical trials. J Rheumatol 2008;35(2):201–5; with permission.)

(Fig. 3).[41] Therefore, improvement in a tender or swollen joint count, even at a 20% level, may nonetheless be associated with further joint damage over time.

Although these observations may not necessarily be regarded as a limitation of a swollen and tender joint count, earlier interpretations that a statistically significant 20% improvement versus placebo indicated that an important treatment effect was not supported by long-term observations. "Tight control" of patient status, with a goal of remission,[52–58] is needed, rather than reduction of swollen and tender joint counts by 20% or even 50%.[52]

JOINT COUNTS ARE NOT AS SENSITIVE AS ULTRASOUND OR MAGNETIC RESONANCE IMAGING IN DETECTING INFLAMMATORY ACTIVITY

Several studies indicate that formal swollen and tender joint counts are not as sensitive as ultrasonography or magnetic resonance imaging (MRI) to detect synovitis. For example, in 644 painful joints of 80 patients with early untreated oligoarthritis involving fewer than 5 joints,[59] synovitis was detected by ultrasound in 150 (33%) of 439 joints that were painful but not swollen, as well as 107 (13%) of 826 joints that were clinically normal (Fig. 4). The findings indicate that patients may have synovitis that is not detectable by clinical examination in a substantial number of affected joints. These studies indicate that tender and swollen joint count may be limited for optimal detection of synovitis or for responses to therapy, explained in part by poor reliability, as discussed earlier.

MOST VISITS TO A RHEUMATOLOGIST INCLUDE A CAREFUL JOINT EXAMINATION, BUT NOT A FORMAL JOINT COUNT

Rheumatologists have been taught extensively that a formal quantitative joint count should be included at each visit of an RA patient.[7] However, a careful joint

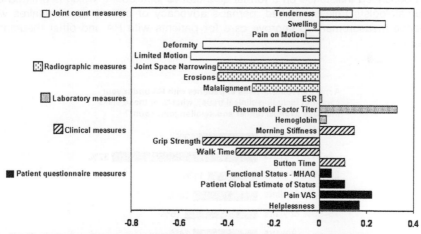

Fig. 3. Changes in measures in 100 patients with rheumatoid arthritis (RA) over 5 years determined by effect sizes, including joint count, radiographic, laboratory, clinical, and patient questionnaire measures. Bars to the right of zero indicate improvement and bars to the left worsening of clinical status. ESR, erythrocyte sedimentation rate; MHAQ, modified health assessment questionnaire; VAS, visual analog scale. (Reproduced from Callahan LF, Pincus T, Huston JW III, et al. Measures of activity and damage in rheumatoid arthritis: depiction of changes and prediction of mortality over five years. Arthritis Care Res 1997;10:381–94; with permission.)

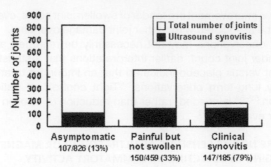

Fig. 4. Prevalence of ultrasound-detected synovitis in joints that were asymptomatic (n = 826), clinically painful but not swollen (n = 425), and clinically synovitic (n = 185). Note detection of ultrasound synovitis in 79% of joints with clinical synovitis but also 33% of joints that were painful but not swollen, and 13% of asymptomatic joints. (*Reproduced from* Wakefield RJ, Green MJ, Marzo-Ortega H, et al. Should oligoarthritis be reclassified? Ultrasound reveals a high prevalence of subclinical disease. Ann Rheum Dis 2004;63:382–5; with permission.)

examination, but not a formal quantitative joint count, is performed at most visits of patients with RA (**Fig. 5**).[60]

Recognition of limitations of the joint count may be of value in efforts to improve quantitative measurement in rheumatic diseases. At this time, both a formal joint count and patient questionnaire are included at all patient visits for clinical trials, but neither is included at most visits in usual care. A patient self-report questionnaire appears to provide as much quantitative information as an *exact* count of the number of swollen and tender joints, and is more easily collected. Therefore, rather than continued insistence on a formal quantitative joint count, which is omitted by rheumatologists unless required, perhaps advocacy of patient questionnaires will advance measurement to improve care for patients with RA and other rheumatic diseases.

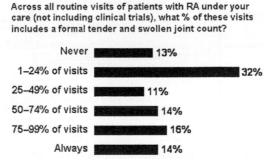

Fig. 5. Self-report responses for performance of formal tender and swollen joint counts, by 550 rheumatologists from 17 European countries. Note: 45% of rheumatologists indicate that fewer than one-fourth of visits include a formal joint count, whereas only 30% include a formal joint count in 75% or more of visits. (*Reproduced from* Pincus T, Segurado OG. Most visits of most patients with rheumatoid arthritis to most rheumatologists do not include a formal quantitative joint count. Ann Rheum Dis 2006;65:820–2; with permission.)

REFERENCES

1. Pincus T. The DAS is the most specific measure, but a patient questionnaire is the most informative measure to assess rheumatoid arthritis. J Rheumatol 2006;33:834–7.
2. Cooperating Clinics Committee of the American Rheumatism Association. A seven-day variability study of 499 patients with peripheral rheumatoid arthritis. Arthritis Rheum 1965;8:302–35.
3. Ritchie DM, Boyle JA, McInnes JM, et al. Clinical studies with an articular index for the assessment of joint tenderness in patients with rheumatoid arthritis. New Series. Q J Med 1968;37:393–406.
4. American Rheumatism Association. Dictionary of the rheumatic diseases. In: Signs and symptoms, vol. I. New York: Contact Associates International; 1982.
5. Decker JL. American Rheumatism Association nomenclature and classification of arthritis and rheumatism. Arthritis Rheum 1983;26:1029–32.
6. Bombardier C, Tugwell P, Sinclair A, et al. Preference for endpoint measures in clinical trials: results of structured workshops. J Rheumatol 1982;9:798–801.
7. Wolfe F, Pincus T, Thompson AK, et al. The assessment of rheumatoid arthritis and the acceptability of self-report questionnaires in clinical practice. Arthritis Care Res 2003;49(1):59–63.
8. Boers M, Tugwell P, Felson DT, et al. World Health Organization and International League of Associations for Rheumatology core endpoints for symptom modifying antirheumatic drugs in rheumatoid arthritis clinical trials. J Rheumatol 1994; 21(Suppl 41):86–9.
9. Felson DT, Anderson JJ, Boers M, et al. The American College of Rheumatology preliminary core set of disease activity measures for rheumatoid arthritis clinical trials. Arthritis Rheum 1993;36:729–40.
10. American College of Rheumatology Committee to Reevaluate Improvement Criteria. A proposed revision to the ACR20: the hybrid measure of American College of Rheumatology response. Arthritis Rheum 2007;57(2):193–202.
11. Goldsmith CH, Smythe HA, Helewa A. Interpretation and power of pooled index. J Rheumatol 1993;20:575–8.
12. van der Heijde DM, van't Hof MA, van Riel PL, et al. Judging disease activity in clinical practice in rheumatoid arthritis: first step in the development of a disease activity score. Ann Rheum Dis 1990;49:916–20.
13. van der Heijde DM, van't Hof M, van Riel PL, van de Putte LB. Development of a disease activity score based on judgment in clinical practice by rheumatologists. J Rheumatol 1993;20:579–81.
14. Aletaha D, Smolen J. The simplified disease activity index (SDAI) and the clinical disease activity index (CDAI): a review of their usefulness and validity in rheumatoid arthritis. Clin Exp Rheumatol 2005;23:S100–8.
15. Lansbury J, Baier HN, McCracken S. Statistical study of variation in systemic and articular indexes. Arthritis Rheum 1962;5:445–56.
16. Eberl DR, Fasching V, Rahlfs V, et al. Repeatability and objectivity of various measurements in rheumatoid arthritis: a comparative study. Arthritis Rheum 1976;19:1278–86.
17. Hanson MT, Keiding S, Lauritzen SL, et al. Clinical assessment of disease activity in rheumatoid arthritis. Scand J Rheumatol 1979;8:101–5.
18. Hart LE, Tugwell P, Buchanan WW, et al. Grading of tenderness as a source of interrater error in the Ritchie articular index. J Rheumatol 1985;12:716–7.
19. Thompson PW, Kirwan JR. Observer variation and the Ritchie articular index. J Rheumatol 1986;13:836–7.

20. Lewis PA, O'Sullivan MM, Rumfeld WR, et al. Significant changes in Ritchie scores. Br J Rheumatol 1988;27:32–6.
21. Klinkhoff AV, Bellamy N, Bombardier C, et al. An experiment in reducing interobserver variability of the examination for joint tenderness. J Rheumatol 1988;15: 492–4.
22. Thompson PW, Kirwan JR, Currey HLF. A comparison of the ability of 28 articular indices to detect an induced flare of joint inflammation in rheumatoid arthritis. Br J Rheumatol 1988;27:375–80.
23. Fuchs HA, Brooks RH, Callahan LF, et al. A simplified twenty-eight joint quantitative articular index in rheumatoid arthritis. Arthritis Rheum 1989;32:531–7.
24. Thompson PW, Hart LE, Goldsmith CH, et al. Comparison of four articular indices for use in clinical trials in rheumatoid arthritis: patient, order and observer variation. J Rheumatol 1991;18:661–5.
25. Bellamy N, Anastassiades TP, Buchanan WW, et al. Rheumatoid arthritis antirheumatic drug trials. 1. Effects of standardization procedures on observer dependent outcome measures. J Rheumatol 1991;18:1893–900.
26. Scott DL, Choy EHS, Greeves A, et al. Standarising joint assessment in rheumatoid arthritis. Clin Rheumatol 1996;15:579–82.
27. Lassere MND, van der Heijde D, Johnson KR, et al. Reliability of measures of disease activity and disease damage in rheumatoid arthritis: implications for smallest detectable difference, minimal clinically important difference, and analysis of treatment effects in randomized controlled trials. J Rheumatol 2001;28(4): 892–903.
28. Sokka T, Pincus T. Quantitative joint assessment in rheumatoid arthritis. Clin Exp Rheumatol 2005;23:S58–62.
29. Pincus T. Limitations of a quantitative swollen and tender joint count to assess and monitor patients with rheumatoid arthritis. Bull NYU Hosp Jt Dis 2008; 66(3):216–23.
30. Tugwell P, Wells G, Strand V, et al. Clinical improvement as reflected in measures of function and health-related quality of life following treatment with leflunomide compared with methotrexate in patients with rheumatoid arthritis: sensitivity and relative efficiency to detect a treatment effect in a twelve-month, placebo-controlled trial. Arthritis Rheum 2000;43(3):506–14.
31. Strand V, Cohen S, Crawford B, et al. Patient-reported outcomes better discriminate active treatment from placebo in randomized controlled trials in rheumatoid arthritis. Rheumatology 2004;43:640–7.
32. Pincus T, Strand V, Koch G, et al. An index of the three core data set patient questionnaire measures distInguishes efficacy of active treatment from placebo as effectively as the American College of Rheumatology 20% response criteria (ACR20) or the disease activity score (DAS) in a rheumatoid arthritis clinical trial. Arthritis Rheum 2003;48(3):625–30.
33. Pincus T, Amara I, Koch GG. Continuous indices of Core Data Set measures in rheumatoid arthritis clinical trials: lower responses to placebo than seen with categorical responses with the American College of Rheumatology 20% criteria. Arthritis Rheum 2005;52:1031–6.
34. Pincus T, Chung C, Segurado OG, et al. An index of patient self-reported outcomes (PRO Index) discriminates effectively between active and control treatment in 4 clinical trials of adalimumab in rheumatoid arthritis. J Rheumatol 2006; 33:2146–52.
35. Pincus T, Bergman MJ, Yazici Y, et al. An index of only patient-reported outcome measures, routine assessment of patient index data 3 (RAPID3), in two abatacept

clinical trials: similar results to disease activity score (DAS28) and other RAPID indices that include physician-reported measures. Rheumatology (Oxford) 2008;47(3):345–9.

36. Pincus T, Amara I, Segurado OG, et al. Relative efficiencies of physician/assessor global estimates and patient questionnaire measures are similar to or greater than joint counts to distinguish adalimumab from control treatments in rheumatoid arthritis clinical trials. J Rheumatol 2008;35(2):201–5.

37. Gotzsche PC. Sensitivity of effect variables in rheumatoid arthritis: a meta-analysis of 130 placebo controlled NSAID trials. J Clin Epidemiol 1990;43:1313–8.

38. Bombardier C, Raboud J. A comparison of health-related quality-of-life measures for rheumatoid arthritis research. The Auranofin Cooperating Group. Control Clin Trials 1991;12:243S–56S.

39. Cohen SB, Strand V, Aguilar D, et al. Patient- versus physician-reported outcomes in rheumatoid arthritis patients treated with recombinant interleukin-1 receptor antagonist (anakinra) therapy. Rheumatology 2004;43(6):704–11.

40. Anderson JJ, Felson DT, Meenan RF, et al. Which traditional measures should be used in rheumatoid arthritis clinical trials? Arthritis Rheum 1989;32:1093–9.

41. Callahan LF, Pincus T, Huston JW III, et al. Measures of activity and damage in rheumatoid arthritis: depiction of changes and prediction of mortality over five years. Arthritis Care Res 1997;10:381–94.

42. Scott DL, Grindulis KA, Struthers GR, et al. Progression of radiological changes in rheumatoid arthritis. Ann Rheum Dis 1984;43:8–17.

43. Pincus T, Callahan LF, Sale WG, et al. Severe functional declines, work disability, and increased mortality in seventy-five rheumatoid arthritis patients studied over nine years. Arthritis Rheum 1984;27:864–72.

44. Hawley DJ, Wolfe F. Sensitivity to change of the Health Assessment Questionnaire (HAQ) and other clinical and health status measures in rheumatoid arthritis: results of short term clinical trials and observational studies versus long term observational studies. Arthritis Care Res 1992;5:130–6.

45. Sharp JT, Wolfe F, Mitchell DM, et al. The progression of erosion and joint space narrowing scores in rheumatoid arthritis during the first twenty-five years of disease. Arthritis Rheum 1991;34:660–8.

46. Egsmose C, Lund B, Borg G, et al. Patients with rheumatoid arthritis benefit from early 2nd line therapy: 5 year followup of a prospective double blind placebo controlled study. J Rheumatol 1995;22:2208–13.

47. Fex E, Jonsson K, Johnson U, et al. Development of radiographic damage during the first 5-6 yr of rheumatoid arthritis. A prospective follow-up study of a Swedish cohort. Br J Rheumatol 1996;35:1106–15.

48. Mulherin D, Fitzgerald O, Bresnihan B. Clinical improvement and radiological deterioration in rheumatoid arthritis: evidence that pathogenesis of synovial inflammation and articular erosion may differ. Br J Rheumatol 1996;35:1263–8.

49. Leirisalo-Repo M, Paimela L, Peltomaa R, et al. Functional and radiological outcome in patients with early RA—a longitudinal observational study [abstract]. Arthritis Rheum 1999;42:S130.

50. Graudal N, Tarp U, Jurik AG, et al. Inflammatory patterns in rheumatoid arthritis estimated by the number of swollen and tender joints, the erythrocyte sedimentation rate, and hemoglobin: longterm course and association to radiographic progression. J Rheumatol 2000;27:47–57.

51. Welsing PMJ, van Gestel AM, Swinkels HL, et al. The relationship between disease activity, joint destruction, and functional capacity over the course of rheumatoid arthritis. Arthritis Rheum 2001;44(9):2009–17.

52. Puolakka K, Kautiainen H, Möttönen T, et al. Early suppression of disease activity is essential for maintenance of work capacity in patients with recent-onset rheumatoid arthritis: five-year experience from the FIN-RACo trial. Arthritis Rheum 2005;52(1):36–41.

53. Puolakka K, Kautiainen H, Mottonen T, et al. Predictors of productivity loss in early rheumatoid arthritis: a 5 year follow up study. Ann Rheum Dis 2005;64:130–3.

54. Pincus T. The case for early intervention in rheumatoid arthritis. J Autoimmun 1992;5(Suppl A):209–26.

55. Pincus T, Callahan LF. The 'side effects' of rheumatoid arthritis: Joint destruction, disability and early mortality. Br J Rheumatol 1993;32(Suppl 1):28–37.

56. Emery P, Salmon M. Early rheumatoid arthritis: time to aim for remission? Ann Rheum Dis 1995;54:944–7.

57. Weinblatt ME. Rheumatoid arthritis: treat now, not later! [editorial]. Ann Intern Med 1996;124:773–4.

58. Pincus T, Gibofsky A, Weinblatt ME. Urgent care and tight control of rheumatoid arthritis as in diabetes and hypertension: better treatments but a shortage of rheumatologists. Arthritis Rheum 2002;46(4):851–4.

59. Wakefield RJ, Green MJ, Marzo-Ortega H, et al. Should oligoarthritis be reclassified? Ultrasound reveals a high prevalence of subclinical disease. Ann Rheum Dis 2004;63:382–5.

60. Pincus T, Segurado OG. Most visits of most patients with rheumatoid arthritis to most rheumatologists do not include a formal quantitative joint count. Ann Rheum Dis 2006;65:820–2.

61. Karim Z, Wakefield RJ, Quinn M, et al. Validation and reproducibility of ultrasonography in the detection of synovitis in the knee: a comparison with arthroscopy and clinical examination. Arthritis Rheum 2004;50:387–94.

62. Kane D, Balint PV, Sturrock RD. Ultrasonography is superior to clinical examination in the detection and localization of knee joint effusion in rheumatoid arthritis. J Rheumatol 2003;30:966–71.

Radiographic Measures to Assess Patients with Rheumatoid Arthritis: Advantages and Limitations

Yusuf Yazici, MD[a], Tuulikki Sokka, MD, PhD[b], Theodore Pincus, MD[a],*

KEYWORDS

- Radiographic scoring • Joint destruction
- Sharp/van der Heijde score • Larsen score

Radiographs present several desirable features for assessment of rheumatoid arthritis (RA) (**Table 1**).[1] Characteristic erosions or symmetric joint space narrowing may provide a finding that is closest to a pathognomonic sign in RA, with few "false-positive" results. The radiograph reflects cumulative damage resulting from uncontrolled inflammation over time. It provides a permanent record, available for comparisons over long periods.

Radiographs were initially scored quantitatively using a global I–IV Steinbrocker grade,[2] which is easily accomplished in standard care but is not sufficiently detailed to recognize changes over time. Many patients may progress substantially while remaining within the same grade. Therefore, excellent detailed quantitative systems have been developed to score radiographs in RA, based on classical systems developed by Larsen and colleagues[3,4] and Sharp and colleagues,[5,6] which are significantly correlated with the Steinbrocker grade. Modifications of the Sharp method have been reported by van der Heijde and colleagues,[7–9] Rau and colleagues,[10] Kaye and colleagues,[11–13] and Genant and colleagues[14,15]; modifications of the Larsen method

---

A version of this article originally appeared in the 21:4 issue of *Best Practice & Research: Clinical Rheumatology*.

[a] Division of Rheumatology, Department of Medicine, New York University School of Medicine and New York University Hospital for Joint Diseases, Room 1608, 301 East 17th Street, New York, NY 10003, USA

[b] Jyväskylä Central Hospital, Jyväskylä, and Medcare Oy, Äänekoski, Finland

* Corresponding author.

E-mail address: tedpincus@gmail.com (T. Pincus).

Rheum Dis Clin N Am 35 (2009) 723–729
doi:10.1016/j.rdc.2009.10.005
0889-857X/09/$ – see front matter © 2009 Elsevier Inc. All rights reserved.

Table 1
Advantages and disadvantages of quantitative radiographic measures in rheumatoid arthritis

Advantages	Disadvantages
Excellent quantitative scoring systems	Quantitative score tedious to perform
Erosions are closest to pathognomonic sign in RA	Less sensitive to detect abnormalities than MRI, ultrasound
Reflect cumulative damage of disease	Radiographic damage has little prognostic value for work disability, death, or even joint replacement

Abbreviation: MRI, magnetic resonance imaging.

have been reported by Larsen,[16] Kaarela and Kautiainen,[17] and Rau and colleagues.[18,19]

At present no simplified systems have been described for quantitation of radiographs in usual clinical care. Rheumatologists generally review radiographs qualitatively, describing whether or not osteopenia, joint space narrowing, and/or erosions are seen. Detailed quantitative radiographic scores are rarely assigned outside of formal clinical research studies. Indeed, most rheumatologists (and radiologists) have no experience in quantitative assessment of radiographs.

Radiography also presents several important limitations as a measure of clinical status in patients with RA (see **Table 1**). Radiographs change slowly in most people, so that at least 6 months to 1 year may be required to assess changes in an individual patient, although it is possible to ascertain statistically significant differences between subjects receiving active versus control treatment in large groups of patients over a period of 12 weeks.

Radiography is less sensitive in recognizing abnormalities than magnetic resonance imaging (MRI) and ultrasonography,[20,21] which are expensive and not available at all treatment centers. Although methods for quantitative scoring of MRI and ultrasonography have been proposed, a consensus does not yet exist regarding optimal scoring. Furthermore, the contemporary approach to patients with RA involves, appropriately, treatment before structural damage, when imaging studies are still normal except for possible osteopenia.

Radiographs are weakly correlated with patient pain and joint tenderness but are correlated significantly with rheumatoid factor and erythrocyte sedimentation rate.[22–24] Two clusters of measures are observed in RA (**Fig. 1**): radiographs are correlated at high levels with duration of disease, laboratory measures, and joint deformity, and at lower levels with age, joint swelling, joint tenderness, functional status, and pain, which in turn are correlated significantly with one another.[22–24]

Radiographs provide optimal documentation of joint destruction but are far weaker predictors of severe outcomes such as work disability, costs, and premature mortality than measures of functional status on patient questionnaires[24–26] (see "Patient Questionnaires in Rheumatoid Arthritis: Advantages and Limitations as a Quantitative, Standardized Scientific Medical History," by Pincus T, et al, in this issue). This observation remains relatively poorly recognized among general physicians and even rheumatologists, many of whom continue to regard radiographic structural change as a most objective measure and therefore of great prognostic importance.

Several reports based on clinical trials indicate that biologic agents in combination with methotrexate are more likely to inhibit radiographic progression than methotrexate alone.[27–29] For example, it was documented in the TEMPO (Trial of Etanercept and Methotrexate With Radiographic Patient Outcome) clinical trial[27] that mean

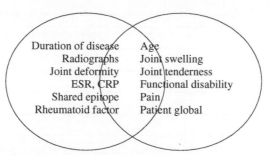

Fig. 1. Two clusters of measures in rheumatoid arthritis. Note that radiographs cluster with joint deformity, erythrocyte sedimentation rate (ESR) and C-reactive protein (CRP), shared epitope, and rheumatoid factor, whereas functional disability clusters with joint tenderness and pain. All measures are correlated with one another. However, measures within each of the two clusters are correlated with one another at higher levels than with measures in the other cluster. Measures in the cluster at the left are more objective than the cluster at the right, and therefore usually are regarded as more significant in long-term outcomes. However, functional disability measures and the cluster at the right provide more significant predictors of severe outcomes of RA, including work disability, premature mortality, and costs than radiographs and measures in the cluster at the left.

radiographic progression according to the Sharp-van der Heijde scores was 3 units over 2 years in patients randomized to methotrexate only compared with 1 unit in patients randomized to etanercept and no progression with even slight improvement in patients randomized to combination therapy with etanercept plus methotrexate (**Fig. 2**). The total Sharp-van der Heijde score involves 448 units, with a smallest detectable difference of 5 units, similar to the minimal clinically important difference of 4.6 units.[30] The scale of the reported data appears greatly exaggerated when compared with a scale with the full range of scores (**Fig. 3**),[31] in which differences between treatment groups are trivial. Furthermore, a probability plot (**Fig. 4**) reveals that about 80% of the patients either had no radiographic progression or improvement

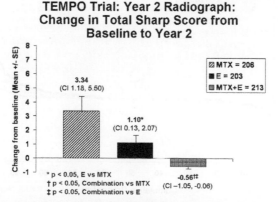

Fig. 2. TEMPO trial. Changes in Sharp/van der Heijde score over 2 years in patients treated with methotrexate, etanercept, and combination of both agents. (*Data from* Klareskog L, van der Heijde D, de Jager JP, et al. Therapeutic effect of the combination of etanercept and methotrexate compared with each treatment alone in patients with rheumatoid arthritis: double-blind randomised controlled trial. Lancet 2004;363:675–81.)

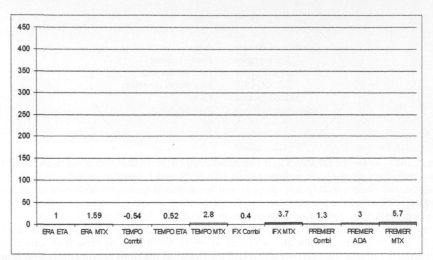

Fig. 3. Changes in Sharp/van der Heijde radiographic scores (0–448) in TEMPO and PREMIER clinical trials. (*Data from* Refs.[27,29,31])

regardless of which treatment was administered and the differences between the 3 treatment groups were demonstrated only in a small fraction of the patients.

A suggestion, based on TEMPO and similar studies, that biologic agents plus methotrexate is superior to methotrexate alone appears to be indicated for groups of patients if 20% to 30% of the patients do not respond to methotrexate and require

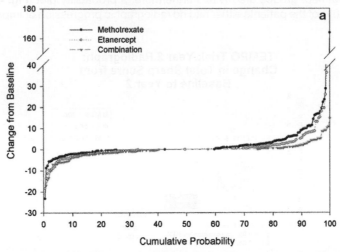

Fig. 4. Change in total Sharp/van der Heijde radiographic scores (0–448) in the TEMPO trial over 2 years. (*Data from* Klareskog L, van der Heijde D, de Jager JP, et al. Therapeutic effect of the combination of etanercept and methotrexate compared with each treatment alone in patients with rheumatoid arthritis: double-blind randomised controlled trial. Lancet 2004;363:675–81.)

a biologic agent to control inflammation. Therefore, the data are valid for patient groups, and a "marketing message" that a biologic agent should be considered for all RA patients is valid. However, 70% to 80% of RA patients experience similar radiographic outcomes regardless of whether they are treated with only methotrexate, with a biologic agent, or with a combination of the two.

Biologic agents are invaluable for the 20% to 30% of patients who have inadequate responses to methotrexate. However, most RA patients need not be treated with a biologic agent; treatment with only methotrexate or methotrexate in combination with a standard disease-modifying antirheumatic drug over 3 to 6 months is appropriate and adequate for 70% to 80% of patients. Very little is lost in radiographic progression over a few months. Furthermore, the impact of radiographic scores is substantially exaggerated in the manner of plotting the data, and radiographic progression itself is less significant than functional status to predict work disability, mortality, and other severe outcomes of RA. Again, biologic agents certainly represent a major advance for the 20% to 30% of patients who require them, but they are not needed in most patients with RA.

Radiographic measurement has been of major importance in the development of concepts concerning the severity of RA and the need for tight control to prevent damage. At the same time, the limitations of radiographs must be recognized in patient management.

REFERENCES

1. Sharp JT. Radiological assessment of joint damage: the premier outcome measure in rheumatoid arthritis. Current status and future potential. In: Wolfe F, Pincus T, editors. Rheumatoid arthritis: pathogenesis, assessment, outcome, and treatment. New York: Marcel Dekker, Inc; 1994. p. 167–89.
2. Steinbrocker O, Traeger CH, Batterman RC. Therapeutic criteria in rheumatoid arthritis. JAMA 1949;140:659–62.
3. Larsen A. A radiological method for grading the severity of rheumatoid arthritis [Academic dissertation]. University of Helsinki. Helsinki; 1974.
4. Larsen A, Dale K, Eek M. Radiographic evaluation of rheumatoid arthritis and related conditions by standard reference films. Acta Radiol Diagn (Stockh) 1977;18:481–91.
5. Sharp JT, Lidsky MD, Collins LC, et al. Methods of scoring the progression of radiologic changes in rheumatoid arthritis: correlation of radiologic, clinical and laboratory abnormalities. Arthritis Rheum 1971;14:706–20.
6. Sharp JT. Scoring radiographic abnormalities in rheumatoid arthritis. J Rheumatol 1989;16:568–9.
7. van der Heijde D. How to read radiographs according to the Sharp/van der Heijde method. J Rheumatol 1999;26:743–5.
8. Landewe R, van der Heijde D. Radiographic progression in rheumatoid arthritis. Clin Exp Rheumatol 2005;23:S63–8.
9. van der Heijde DM, van Leeuwen MA, van Riel PL, et al. Biannual radiographic assessments of hands and feet in a three-year prospective followup of patients with early rheumatoid arthritis. Arthritis Rheum 1992;35:26–34.
10. Rau R, Wassenberg S, Herborn G, et al. A new method of scoring radiographic change in rheumatoid arthritis. J Rheumatol 1998;25:2094–107.
11. Nance EP Jr, Kaye JJ, Callahan LF, et al. Observer variation in quantitative assessment of rheumatoid arthritis: part I. Scoring erosions and joint space narrowing. Invest Radiol 1986;21:922–7.

12. Kaye JJ, Nance EP, Callahan LF, et al. Observer variation in quantitative assessment of rheumatoid arthritis: part II. A simplified scoring system. Invest Radiol 1987;22:41–6.

13. Kaye JJ, Callahan LF, Nance EP Jr, et al. Bony ankylosis in rheumatoid arthritis: associations with longer duration and greater severity of disease. Invest Radiol 1987;22:303–9.

14. Genant HK. Methods of assessing radiographic change in rheumatoid arthritis. Am J Med 1983;75(Suppl 6A):35–47.

15. Genant HK, Jiang Y, Peterfy C, et al. Assessment of rheumatoid arthritis using a modified scoring method on digitized and original radiographs. Arthritis Rheum 1998;41:1583–90.

16. Larsen A. How to apply Larsen score in evaluating radiographs of rheumatoid arthritis in long-term studies? J Rheumatol 1995;22:1974–5.

17. Kaarela K, Kautiainen H. Continuous progression of radiological destruction in seropositive rheumatoid arthritis. J Rheumatol 1997;24:1285–7.

18. Rau R, Herborn G. A modified version of Larsen's scoring method to assess radiologic changes in rheumatoid arthritis. J Rheumatol 1995;22:1976–82.

19. Rau R, Wassenberg S, Herborn G, et al. Identification of radiologic healing phenomena in patients with rheumatoid arthritis. J Rheumatol 2001;28:2608–15.

20. Wakefield RJ, Kong KO, Conaghan PG, et al. The role of ultrasonography and magnetic resonance imaging in early rheumatoid arthritis. Clin Exp Rheumatol 2003;21:S42–9.

21. Klarlund M, Ostergaard M, Jensen KE, et al. Magnetic resonance imaging, radiography, and scintigraphy of the finger joints: one year follow up of patients with early arthritis. The TIRA Group 3. Ann Rheum Dis 2000;59:521–8.

22. Pincus T, Callahan LF, Brooks RH, et al. Self-report questionnaire scores in rheumatoid arthritis compared with traditional physical, radiographic, and laboratory measures. Ann Intern Med 1989;110:259–66.

23. Sokka T, Kankainen A, Hannonen P. Scores for functional disability in patients with rheumatoid arthritis are correlated at higher levels with pain scores than with radiographic scores. Arthritis Rheum 2000;43:386–9.

24. Pincus T, Sokka T. Quantitative measures and indices to assess rheumatoid arthritis in clinical trials and clinical care. Rheum Dis Clin North Am 2004;30: 725–51.

25. Pincus T, Callahan LF. What is the natural history of rheumatoid arthritis? Rheum Dis Clin North Am 1993;19:123–51.

26. Pincus T, Sokka T. Quantitative measures for assessing rheumatoid arthritis in clinical trials and clinical care. Best Pract Res Clin Rheumatol 2003;17: 753–81.

27. Klareskog L, van der Heijde D, de Jager JP, et al. Therapeutic effect of the combination of etanercept and methotrexate compared with each treatment alone in patients with rheumatoid arthritis: double-blind randomised controlled trial. Lancet 2004;363:675–81.

28. StClair EW, van der Heijde DM, Smolen JS, et al. Combination of infliximab and methotrexate therapy for early rheumatoid arthritis: a randomized, controlled trial. Arthritis Rheum 2004;50:3432–43.

29. Breedveld FC, Weisman MH, Kavanaugh AF, et al. The PREMIER study: a multicenter, randomized, double-blind clinical trial of combination therapy with adalimumab plus methotrexate versus methotrexate alone or adalimumab alone in patients with early, aggressive rheumatoid arthritis who had not had previous methotrexate treatment. Arthritis Rheum 2006;54:26–37.

30. Bruynesteyn K, van der HD, Boers M, et al. Determination of the minimal clinically important difference in rheumatoid arthritis joint damage of the Sharp/van der Heijde and Larsen/Scott scoring methods by clinical experts and comparison with the smallest detectable difference. Arthritis Rheum 2002;46:913–20.
31. Yazici Y, Yazici H. Trial of etanercept and methotrexate with radiographic and patient outcomes two-year clinical and radiographic results: comment on the article by van der Heijde et al. Arthritis Rheum 2006;54:3061–2.

Laboratory Tests to Assess Patients with Rheumatoid Arthritis: Advantages and Limitations

Theodore Pincus, MD[a],*, Tuulikki Sokka, MD, PhD[b]

KEYWORDS

- Erythrocyte sedimentation rate • C-reactive protein
- Cyclic citrullinated peptide • Rheumatoid factor

Laboratory tests provide the most definitive information in diagnosis, management, prognosis, and documentation of course of many diseases, according to a biomedical model.[1] The discovery in the 1940s of rheumatoid factor (RF)[2,3] in most patients with rheumatoid arthritis (RA) and antinuclear antibodies (ANA)[4] in almost all patients with systemic lupus erythematosus (SLE) led to hopes that laboratory tests could serve as "gold standard" measures in rheumatic diseases, analogous to serum cholesterol, creatinine, glucose, hemoglobin A1C, and other tests.

Most patients (and many physicians) look to laboratory tests as the most important information from a medical visit. Changes in values for laboratory tests reflect the pathophysiology of disease far more than other measures such as a tender joint count or patient questionnaire score for pain.

Reduction of levels of RF or erythrocyte sedimentation rate (ESR) in RA (or anti-DNA antibodies in SLE) appears to reflect control of mechanisms thought to result in organ damage.

Most patients with RA do have positive tests for RF and antibodies to cyclic citrullinated peptides (anti-CCP).[5–8] RF is included in classification criteria for RA,[9]

Supported in part by a research grant from Bristol Myers-Squibb, and EVO grants of the Rheumatism Foundation Hospital, Heinola, Finland.

A version of this article originally appeared in the 21:4 issue of *Best Practice & Research: Clinical Rheumatology*.

[a] Division of Rheumatology, Department of Medicine, New York University School of Medicine and NYU Hospital for Joint Diseases, Room 1608, 301 East 17th Street, New York, NY 10003, USA

[b] Jyväskylä Central Hospital, Jyväskylä, and Medcare Oy, Äänekoski, Finland

* Corresponding author.

E-mail address: tedpincus@gmail.com (T. Pincus).

and anti-CCP is being considered for revised criteria. A meta-analysis indicated a positive likelihood ratio of 12.5 and odds ratio (OR) of 16.1 to 39.0 for RA in 37 studies of anti-CCP antibodies, compared with a positive likelihood ratio of 4.9 and OR for RA of 1.2 to 8.7 in 50 studies of RF (**Table 1**).[8]

Most patients with RA also have an elevated ESR and C-reactive protein (CRP).[10] An abnormal ESR or CRP often provides an inclusion criterion for clinical trials.[11] An ESR less than 30 mm/h in a woman and less than 20 mm/h in a man is required to meet American College of Rheumatology (ACR) remission criteria.[12] Reductions in ESR and CRP are seen in groups of patients in all successful clinical trials of RA therapies that indicate efficacy of an active treatment compared with a control treatment.

As noted in Pincus T, Yazici Y, Sokka T., "Complexities in Assessment of Rheumatoid Arthritis: Absence of a Single Gold Standard Measure," in this issue, however, no rheumatology blood test is 100% positive in any rheumatic disease and 100% negative in all normal individuals. Anti-CCP is found in 67% and RF in 69% of patients with RA (see **Table 1**).[8] Therefore, more than 30% of patients have negative tests for these serologic markers. ESR or CRP is normal in about 40% of patients with RA, reported initially in 1994 by Wolfe and Michaud[13] from Wichita, Kansas, and confirmed recently at two sites, one in Nashville, Tennessee, and the other in Jyväskylä, Finland (**Table 2**).[10] Mean ESR levels have declined from 50 mm/h in RA cohorts from 1954 to 1980, to 41 mm/h from 1981 to 1984, to 35 mm/h after 1985.[14] Furthermore, while a decline in ESR or CRP is seen concomitantly with clinical improvement in many patients and in groups of patients in clinical trials, ESR and CRP tend to remain at similar levels in many other individual patients, even with clinical improvement.[15]

The above data indicate that a negative test (ie, false-negative result) is seen in more than 30% of people with a diagnosis of RA for RF, anti-CCP, ESR, or CRP. In addition, false-positive results are seen in people who have other inflammatory diseases, and in some who may not have any inflammatory rheumatic disease at all. In population surveys, about 1% of the normal population has a positive test for RF.[16] Therefore, because the prevalence of RA is 0.5% in most studies,[17,18] a positive test for RF is seen in as many people who do not have RA as in people who have this disease.[16] Obviously, tests for RF are not ordered in all people, but the prevalence of musculoskeletal symptoms in the population may range from 15% to 45%,[17,19,20] including fibromyalgia in 5%.[21,22] Many people with RF have fibromyalgia—probably at least as many as have RA—based on population data.

Table 1
Meta-analysis concerning anti-CCP antibodies and RF in patients with RA and healthy individuals in the general population

	Anti-CCP	RF
Number of studies	37	50
Positive likelihood ratio	12.5	4.9
Odds ratio for RA	16.1–39.0	1.2–8.7
Sensitivity	67%	69%
Specificity	95%	85%
% of RA patients with negative test	33%	31%
% of general population with positive test	5%	15%

Data from Nishimura K, Sugiyama D, Kogata Y, et al. Meta-analysis: diagnostic accuracy of anticyclic citrullinated peptide antibody and rheumatoid factor for rheumatoid arthritis. Ann Intern Med 2007;146:797–808.

Table 2
Number (%) at presentation of rheumatoid arthritis patients with ESR < or ≥28 mm/h in Jyväskylä, Finland, and in Nashville, Tennessee, compared with CRP < or ≥10 in: 1744 patients in Jyväskylä and 170 patients in Nashville

Jyväskylä, Finland

CRP	ESR		Total
	≥28 mm/h	<28 mm/h	
≥10 mg/L	775 (44%)	202 (12%)	977 (56%)
<10 mg/L	199 (11%)	568 (33%)	767 (44%)
Total	974 (56%)	770 (44%)	1744 (100%)

Nashville, Tennessee, USA

CRP	ESR		Total
	≥28 mm/h	<28 mm/h	
≥10 mg/L	48 (28%)	22 (13%)	70 (41%)
<10 mg/L	29 (17%)	71 (42%)	100 (59%)
Total	77 (45%)	93 (55%)	170 (100%)

Data from Sokka T, Pincus T. Erythrocyte sedimentation rate, C-reactive protein, or rheumatoid factor are normal at presentation in 35%–45% of patients with rheumatoid arthritis seen between 1980 and 2004: analyses from Finland and the United States. J Rheumatol 2009;36:1387–90.

The data noted concerning the prevalence of positive laboratory tests in patients with RA are derived from rheumatology treatment centers. Patients must be referred to these settings by primary care physicians, and referral may be less likely if these tests are normal. More than a few patients report that a physician has told them "Your test for rheumatoid arthritis was negative." Observations that more than 30% of patients with RA have negative tests for RF or anti-CCP, and 40% have normal ESR or CRP, may be underestimates.

Another important limitation of laboratory tests is that they often are not available at the time at which a clinical decision is made. A clinician may arrange for a laboratory test in advance of a visit, or contact a patient at a later date, but these practices do not occur in most clinical settings. Therefore, clinical decisions usually are made without laboratory data.

Of course, laboratory research is essential to provide new insights into pathogenesis and new treatments for rheumatic diseases. In usual clinical care, however, laboratory tests often have limited sensitivity and sensitivity, with high levels of false-positive and false-negative results. Physicians and patients may attribute disproportionate importance to laboratory tests in rheumatic diseases.

REFERENCES

1. Engel GL. The need for a new medical model: a challenge for biomedicine. Science 1977;196:129–36.
2. Waaler E. On the occurrence of a factor in human serum activating the specific agglutination of sheep blood corpuscles. Acta Pathol Microbiol Scand 1940;17:172–8.
3. Rose HM, Ragan C, Pearce E, et al. Differential agglutination of normal and sensitized sheep erythrocytes by sera of patients with rheumatoid arthritis. Proc Soc Exp Biol Med 1948;68:1–6.
4. Hargraves MM, Richmond H, Morton R. Presentation of two bone marrow elements: the tart cell and L.E. cell. Mayo Clin Proc 1948;23:25–8.

5. Schellekens GA, de Jong BAW, van den Hoogen FHJ, et al. Citrulline is an essential constituent of antigenic determinants recognized by rheumatoid arthritis-specific autoantibodies. J Clin Invest 1998;101:273–81.

6. van Gaalen FA, Linn-Rasker SP, van Venrooij WJ, et al. Autoantibodies to cyclic citrullinated peptides predict progression to rheumatoid arthritis in patients with undifferentiated arthritis: a prospective cohort study. Arthritis Rheum 2004;50: 709–15.

7. Riedemann JP, Muñoz S, Kavanaugh A. The use of second generation anti-CCP antibody (anti-CCP2) testing in rheumatoid arthritis—a systematic review. Clin Exp Rheumatol 2005;23:S69–76.

8. Nishimura K, Sugiyama D, Kogata Y, et al. Meta-analysis: diagnostic accuracy of anti-cyclic citrullinated peptide antibody and rheumatoid factor for rheumatoid arthritis. Ann Intern Med 2007;146:797–808.

9. Arnett FC, Edworthy SM, Bloch DA, et al. The American Rheumatism Association 1987 revised criteria for the classification of rheumatoid arthritis. Arthritis Rheum 1988;31:315–24.

10. Sokka T, Pincus T. Erythrocyte sedimentation rate, C-reactive protein, or rheumatoid factor are normal at presentation in 35%–45% of patients with rheumatoid arthritis seen between 1980 and 2004: analyses from Finland and the United States. J Rheumatol 2009;36:1387–90.

11. Sokka T, Pincus T. Most patients receiving routine care for rheumatoid arthritis in 2001 did not meet inclusion criteria for most recent clinical trials or American College of Rheumatology criteria for remission. J Rheumatol 2003;30:1138–46.

12. Pinals RS, Masi AT, Larsen RA, et al. Preliminary criteria for clinical remission in rheumatoid arthritis. Arthritis Rheum 1981;24:1308–15.

13. Wolfe F, Michaud K. The clinical and research significance of the erythrocyte sedimentation rate. J Rheumatol 1994;21:1227–37.

14. Abelson B, Sokka T, Pincus T. Declines in erythrocyte sedimentation rates in patients with rheumatoid arthritis over the second half of the 20th century. J Rheumatol 2009;36:1596–9.

15. Wolfe F, Pincus T. The level of inflammation in rheumatoid arthritis is determined early and remains stable over the long-term course of the illness. J Rheumatol 2001;28:1817–24.

16. Pincus T. A pragmatic approach to cost-effective use of laboratory tests and imaging procedures in patients with musculoskeletal symptoms. Prim Care 1993;20:795–814.

17. Helmick CG, Felson DT, Lawrence RC, et al. Estimates of the prevalence of arthritis and other rheumatic conditions in the United States. Part I. Arthritis Rheum 2008;58:15–25.

18. Silman AJ, Pearson JE. Epidemiology and genetics of rheumatoid arthritis. Arthritis Res 2002;4(Suppl 3):S265–72.

19. Mäkelä M, Heliövaara M, Sievers K, et al. Musculoskeletal disorders as determinants of disability in Finns aged 30 years or more. J Clin Epidemiol 1993;46: 549–59.

20. Lawrence RC, Felson DT, Helmick CG, et al. Estimates of the prevalence of arthritis and other rheumatic conditions in the United States. Part II. Arthritis Rheum 2008;58:26–35.

21. Croft P, Rigby AS, Boswell R, et al. The prevalence of chronic widespread pain in the general population. J Rheumatol 1993;20:710–3.

22. Wolfe F, Ross K, Anderson J, et al. The prevalence and characteristics of fibromyalgia in the general population. Arthritis Rheum 1995;38:19–28.

Patient Questionnaires in Rheumatoid Arthritis: Advantages and Limitations as a Quantitative, Standardized Scientific Medical History

Theodore Pincus, MD[a],*, Yusuf Yazici, MD[a], Martin J. Bergman, MD[b]

KEYWORDS

- HAQ (health assessment questionnaire)
- MDHAQ (multidimensional health assessment questionnaire)
- Rheumatoid arthritis • Patient self-report questionnaires

The standard approach to a patient with any disease involves collection of four types of information: from a patient history, physical examination, laboratory tests, and imaging studies. In many chronic diseases, objective "gold standard" measures such as blood pressure, cholesterol, and bone densitometry provide most of the information to guide therapy (see "Complexities in Assessment of Rheumatoid

A version of this article originally appeared in the 21:4 issue of *Best Practice & Research: Clinical Rheumatology*.

Supported in part by grants from the Arthritis Foundation, the Jack C. Massey Foundation, Bristol-Myers Squibb, Amgen.

[a] Division of Rheumatology, Department of Medicine, New York University School of Medicine and NYU Hospital for Joint Diseases, Room 1608, 301 East 17th Street, New York, NY 10003, USA

[b] Division of Rheumatology, Taylor Hospital, Ridley Park, PA, USA

* Corresponding author. Division of Rheumatology, New York University Hospital for Joint Diseases, Room 1608, 301 East 17th Street, New York, NY 10003.

E-mail address: tedpincus@gmail.com (T. Pincus).

Rheum Dis Clin N Am 35 (2009) 735–743

doi:10.1016/j.rdc.2009.10.009

0889-857X/09/$ – see front matter © 2009 Elsevier Inc. All rights reserved.

rheumatic.theclinics.com

Arthritis: Absence of a Single Gold Standard Measure," by Pincus and colleagues, in this issue). By contrast, in patients with inflammatory rheumatic diseases, information from a patient history is considerably more prominent in guiding assessment, management, and prognosis.

Patient history data can be recorded as standardized, quantitative scientific data using validated self-report questionnaires to guide clinical care complemented by objective measures (**Box 1**).[1] Patient questionnaires address the primary concerns of patients and their families. Patient questionnaires are correlated significantly with objective joint counts, laboratory tests, and radiographic scores.[2]

In clinical trials, patient questionnaire scores indicate lesser improvement than swollen and tender joint counts in patients who receive placebo or control treatments.[3] For example, in a trial of leflunomide or methotrexate or placebo,[3] placebo treatment resulted in improvement of 21% for swollen joint count, 20% for tender joint count, 12% for physician global estimate of status, and 12% for patient global estimate of status, but worsening of status of 20% for pain, 9% for physical function, and 22% for erythrocyte sedimentation rate (ESR) (**Fig. 1**).

Patient questionnaires are effective in clinical research, with capacity to distinguish active from control treatments in clinical trials of methotrexate,[3] leflunomide,[3] anakinra,[4] adalimumab,[5] and abatacept,[6] in the same range as swollen and tender joint counts or laboratory tests. For example, in four adalimumab clinical trials,[5] physical function scores had higher relative efficiencies compared with tender joint count in capacity to distinguish patients who received adalimumab versus control treatments in three of eight comparisons, pain in three of eight comparisons, patient global estimate in four of eight comparisons, C-reactive protein (CRP) in four of eight comparisons, and swollen joint count in two of eight comparisons.

An index of only the three patient self-report RA core data set measures—physical function, pain, and patient global estimate—routine assessment of patient index data

---

Box 1
Advantages and limitations of patient self-report questionnaires

Advantages

    Address the primary concerns of patients and their families

    Significantly correlated with joint counts, ESR, radiographic scores, physical measures

    Distinguish active from control treatments in clinical trials in the same range as DAS28 and CDAI

    More reproducible and less likely to improve with placebo than traditional joint counts

    Useful to monitor patient status over time

    Predict work disability, costs, joint replacement, and premature death better than traditional joint counts, radiographs, and laboratory tests

Limitations

    Specialized questionnaires are too cumbersome for usual clinical care—need short questionnaires

    Nonspecific—may improve due to developments unrelated to RA

    Subject to cultural differences (eg, pain scores highest in Latino patients and lowest in Asian patients)

    Must be translated into various languages

    May be subject to gaming by certain patients to give desired answers

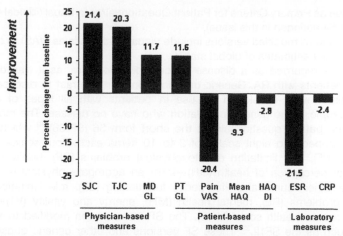

Fig. 1. Mean of the individual percentage changes from baseline in patient- and physician-reported measures for placebo patients at 6 months. The arrow to the left denotes improvement, indicating that deterioration in pain, physical function, and laboratory assessments were reported with placebo treatment. CRP data exclude one outlier subject in the placebo group (percentage change more than 2 SD from the mean). *Abbreviations:* CRP, C-reactive protein; ESR, erythrocyte sedimentation rate; HAQ, health assessment questionnaire; HAQ DI, HAQ disability index; MDGL, physician global estimate of status; PTGL, patient global estimate of status; SJC, swollen joint count. TJC, tender joint count; VAS, visual analog scale. (*Reproduced from* Strand V, Cohen S, Crawford B, et al. Patient-reported outcomes better discriminate active treatment from placebo in randomized controlled trials in rheumatoid arthritis. Rheumatology 2004;43:640–47; with permission.)

(RAPID3), without joint counts, is correlated significantly with the disease activity score 28 (DAS28) and clinical disease activity index (CDAI), indices that do include joint counts, in clinical trials[7] and in clinical settings (see "RAPID3, an Index to Assess and Monitor Patients with Rheumatoid Arthritis, Without Formal Joint Counts: Similar Results to DAS28 and CDAI in Clinical Trials and Clinical Care," by Pincus and colleagues, in this issue).[8,9] Patient questionnaires—not joint counts, radiographic scores, or laboratory tests—provide the most significant predictors of all severe long-term outcomes in patients with RA, including functional status,[10,11] work disability,[12–14] costs,[15] joint replacement surgery,[16] and premature death.[10,17–24] Patient questionnaires are useful to monitor patient status in usual clinical care over time, with almost no effort on the part of the physician and staff if distributed by the receptionist in the infrastructure of office practice.[25,26]

The most prominent questionnaire used to assess patients with RA is the health assessment questionnaire (HAQ).[27] The HAQ includes a scale of 20 activities of daily living (ADL), in eight categories of two or three ADL per category, to assess functional disability, with four patient response options: without any difficulty = 0; with some difficulty = 1; with much difficulty = 2; unable to do = 3.

Several modifications have been made to the HAQ over the years for use in standard clinical care, including a modified HAQ (MHAQ)[28] with eight activities, one from each category on the HAQ,[28] an HAQ II that has superior scaling properties compared with the HAQ and other HAQ derivatives,[29] and a multidimensional HAQ (MDHAQ)[30,31] that adds two complex activities: "Are you able to walk 2 miles or 3 km?" and "Are you able to participate in recreation and sports as you would like?" (see "The HAQ Compared with the MDHAQ: "Keep It Simple, Stupid" (KISS), with Feasibility and

Clinical Value as Primary Criteria for Patient Questionnaires in Usual Clinical Care," by Pincus and Swearingen in this issue).

The HAQ and all modified versions include visual analog scales (VAS) to quantitate pain and patient estimates of global status.

The HAQ is regarded as a disease-specific questionnaire, as it was developed to assess patients with RA. Generic questionnaires, in contrast to disease-specific questionnaires, were developed for use in patients with all types of diseases, including people in the general population who have no disease. The most widely used generic patient questionnaire is the short form 36 (SF-36),[32] which includes 36 items grouped into eight scales of 2 to 10 items each. Four scales—physical functioning (PF), role limitation due to physical problems (RP), bodily pain (BP), and general perception of health (GH)—form an aggregate physical health scale (PHS). The other four scales—for social functioning (SF), role limitation due to emotional problems (RE), mental health (MH), energy and vitality (VT)—form an aggregate mental health scale (MHS). The SF-36 has been modified to shortened versions such as the SF12.[33] These SF versions and other generic questionnaires can be used to compare the impacts of a specific rheumatic disease versus other rheumatic diseases, as well as nonrheumatic chronic diseases such as congestive heart failure or lymphoma, on quality of life. It appears, however, that the HAQ and its derivatives also can function as a largely generic questionnaire for people with many types of diseases.[34]

Additional questionnaires are available to assess functional disability, such as the arthritis impact measurement scales (AIMS),[35] and quality of life, such as the European quality of life index (EuroQoL).[36] More detailed questionnaires beyond simple VAS are available to assess pain, such as the McGill pain questionnaire,[37] and fatigue.[38] An individualized measure such as the McMaster-Toronto arthritis patient preference questionnaire (MACTAR) index[39] or the patient evaluation technique (PET) index[40] is designed to be customized to each individual patient.

Additional disease-specific questionnaires for rheumatic diseases other than RA have been developed, such as the Western Ontario McMaster osteoarthritis index (WOMAC)[41] and fibromyalgia impact questionnaire (FIQ).[42] A recent development involves individualized questionnaires using computer-assisted technology (CAT), in which a response to one question triggers appropriate additional questions to reduce redundancy and give a standard score for physical function based on different items.[43]

Patient questionnaire data have been used in lieu of standard patient visits to monitor patients with RA in stable clinical status.[44] This strategy may be promising for certain patients, in view of shortage of rheumatologists in most countries, which is projected to continue and perhaps worsen.[45] At a clinical encounter, however, while a patient questionnaire provides important components of a standardized patient history, a patient questionnaire cannot be viewed as a substitute for a standard medical evaluation with further patient history, physical examination, laboratory tests, and imaging studies.

As discussed at greater length elsewhere (see "How to Collect an MDHAQ to Provide Rheumatology Vital Signs (Function, Pain, Global Status, and RAPID3 Scores) in the Infrastructure of Rheumatology Care, Including Some Misconceptions Regarding the MDHAQ," by Pincus and colleagues, in this issue), it is important that health professionals allow patients to complete self-report questionnaires by themselves, which improves accuracy and reliability by including only one observer. Furthermore, the most effective strategy to ensure completion of patient questionnaires is for the receptionist to ask each patient to complete a simple questionnaire at each visit. It is desirable for the physician to have available patient questionnaire scores at the time the patient is seen, which requires completion in a waiting room area.

Patient questionnaires do have limitations (see **Box 1**), as is the case for all clinical measures. Many patient questionnaires are too cumbersome for standard clinical care and are used only in research, contributing to a situation in which most rheumatologists do not include patient questionnaires in their patient care.[46,47] Questionnaires designed for clinical care on a regular basis differ from research questionnaires (see "Complex Measures and Indices for Clinical Research Compared with Simple Patient Questionnaires to Assess Function, Pain, and Global Estimates as Rheumatology "Vital Signs" for Usual Clinical Care," by Pincus and colleagues, in this issue). Clinicians who include questionnaires designed for clinical care in the infrastructure of care[25,26] (including the authors) find that this practice saves time, allows shorter or more efficient visits, with an opportunity to focus on patient concerns rather than gathering factual information. The primary reasons cited by clinicians for non-use of questionnaires are that it "takes too much staff time" or "the staff will not cooperate," impressions generally derived from lengthy patient questionnaires designed for clinical research (see "How to Collect an MDHAQ to Provide Rheumatology Vital Signs (Function, Pain, Global Status, and RAPID3 Scores) in the Infrastructure of Rheumatology Care, Including Some Misconceptions Regarding the MDHAQ," by Pincus and colleagues, in this issue).

Patient questionnaires are not as specific to assess the degree of inflammatory activity as measures such as swollen joint counts in RA or muscle enzymes in polymyositis. A patient's pain score may improve or decline considerably because of developments other than direct changes of inflammatory status (eg, a score may improve on the basis of good news, but may be higher [more pain] as a result of severe back pain or an injury). This phenomenon emphasizes that any measure, whether a questionnaire score, laboratory test, or radiographic score, must be interpreted by a clinician in formulating clinical decisions.

Patient questionnaire scores may appear to be more affected by joint damage than swollen and tender joint counts, or laboratory tests of acute-phase reactants such as ESR and CRP, and hence less sensitive to recognize control of inflammation.[48] Questionnaire scores, however, are as responsive to distinguish active from control treatments in clinical trials as joint counts and laboratory tests, as noted previously. Therefore, it is likely that joint counts may be affected by damage as much as questionnaire scores. For example, a swollen metacarpal phalangeal (MCP) joint that is affected by subluxation is considerably less likely to show resolution of swelling with active treatment than a nonsubluxed swollen MCP joint.

Patient questionnaires are subject to cultural differences; for example, Latino patients have highest pain scores compared with Caucasians and African Americans, while Asian patients have lowest pain scores.[49] These cultural influences are not seen in assessment of physical function using performance measures such as grip strength and walking time.[50,51] Physical tests, however, are rarely used any longer despite their documented value in monitoring patient prognosis.[52]

Patient questionnaires must be translated into different languages. Ironically, a need to translate questionnaires may provide a potential advantage, in that a translated version may be used rather than a translator. Recognition of a pattern on an MDHAQ allows self-report to provide "translation" that often may be more accurate than information obtained through a translator. As noted previously, one advantage of a patient questionnaire is that it includes only a single observer (ie, the patient), which has been found more accurate than two observers (ie, a health professional and the patient).[27]

The addition of a translator as yet a third observer may reduce reliability of the information further, which may be overcome in part by a self-report questionnaire.

Patient questionnaires may hypothetically be subject to "gaming" on the part of a patient, who might regard certain responses as likely to engender a desired result. For example, a patient seeking work disability may indicate severe problems with physical function, pain, and global status, which may exaggerate the problems, while a patient who is trying to gain employment may underestimate such problems. This type of hypothetical problem rarely is seen in clinical care (health professionals appear more likely than patients to tailor responses to what appears desirable), but may develop into more of a problem with further use of patient questionnaires.

In conclusion, because assessment and monitoring of patients with rheumatic diseases depends more on information from a patient than from laboratory tests, patient history information should be recorded as standardized scientific quantitative data on a patient questionnaire. A simple patient questionnaire that has been found useful in patients with all rheumatic diseases provides a promising approach to introduce quantitative measurement to standard clinical rheumatology care.

REFERENCES

1. Pincus T, Yazici Y, Sokka T. Quantitative measures of rheumatic diseases for clinical research versus standard clinical care: differences, advantages, and limitations. Best Pract Res Clin Rheumatol 2007;21:601–28.
2. Pincus T, Callahan LF, Brooks RH, et al. Self-report questionnaire scores in rheumatoid arthritis compared with traditional physical, radiographic, and laboratory measures. Ann Intern Med 1989;110:259–66.
3. Strand V, Cohen S, Crawford B, et al. Patient-reported outcomes better discriminate active treatment from placebo in randomized controlled trials in rheumatoid arthritis. Rheumatology 2004;43:640–7.
4. Cohen SB, Strand V, Aguilar D, et al. Patient- versus physician-reported outcomes in rheumatoid arthritis patients treated with recombinant interleukin-1 receptor antagonist (anakinra) therapy. Rheumatology 2004;43:704–11.
5. Pincus T, Amara I, Segurado OG, et al. Relative efficiencies of physician/assessor global estimates and patient questionnaire measures are similar to or greater than joint counts to distinguish adalimumab from control treatments in rheumatoid arthritis clinical trials. J Rheumatol 2008;35:201–5.
6. Wells G, Li T, Maxwell L, et al. Responsiveness of patient reported outcomes including fatigue, sleep quality, activity limitation, and quality of life following treatment with abatacept for rheumatoid arthritis. Ann Rheum Dis 2008;67: 260–5.
7. Pincus T, Bergman MJ, Yazici Y, et al. An index of only patient-reported outcome measures, routine assessment of patient index data 3 (RAPID3), in two abatacept clinical trials: similar results to disease activity score (DAS28) and other RAPID indices that include physician-reported measures. Rheumatology (Oxford) 2008;47:345–9.
8. Wolfe F, Michaud K, Pincus T. A composite disease activity scale for clinical practice, observational studies and clinical trials: the patient activity scale (PAS/PAS-II). J Rheumatol 2005;32:2410–5.
9. Pincus T, Swearingen CJ, Bergman M, et al. RAPID3 (routine assessment of patient index data 3), a rheumatoid arthritis index without formal joint counts for routine care: proposed severity categories compared to DAS and CDAI categories. J Rheumatol 2008;35:2136–47.

10. Pincus T, Callahan LF, Sale WG, et al. Severe functional declines, work disability, and increased mortality in seventy-five rheumatoid arthritis patients studied over nine years. Arthritis Rheum 1984;27:864–72.
11. Wolfe F, Cathey MA. The assessment and prediction of functional disability in rheumatoid arthritis. J Rheumatol 1991;18:1298–306.
12. Callahan LF, Bloch DA, Pincus T. Identification of work disability in rheumatoid arthritis: Physical, radiographic and laboratory variables do not add explanatory power to demographic and functional variables. J Clin Epidemiol 1992; 45:127–38.
13. Wolfe F, Hawley DJ. The long-term outcomes of rheumatoid arthritis: work disability: a prospective 18-year study of 823 patients. J Rheumatol 1998;25:2108–17.
14. Sokka T, Kautiainen H, Möttönen T, et al. Work disability in rheumatoid arthritis 10 years after the diagnosis. J Rheumatol 1999;26:1681–5.
15. Lubeck DP, Spitz PW, Fries JF, et al. A multicenter study of annual health service utilization and costs in rheumatoid arthritis. Arthritis Rheum 1986;29:488–93.
16. Wolfe F, Zwillich SH. The long-term outcomes of rheumatoid arthritis: a 23-year prospective, longitudinal study of total joint replacement and its predictors in 1600 patients with rheumatoid arthritis. Arthritis Rheum 1998;41:1072–82.
17. Wolfe F, Kleinheksel SM, Cathey MA, et al. The clinical value of the Stanford health assessment questionnaire functional disability Index in patients with rheumatoid arthritis. J Rheumatol 1988;15:1480–8.
18. Leigh JP, Fries JF. Mortality predictors among 263 patients with rheumatoid arthritis. J Rheumatol 1991;18:1307–12.
19. Pincus T, Brooks RH, Callahan LF. Prediction of long-term mortality in patients with rheumatoid arthritis according to simple questionnaire and joint count measures. Ann Intern Med 1994;120:26–34.
20. Callahan LF, Cordray DS, Wells G, et al. Formal education and five-year mortality in rheumatoid arthritis: mediation by helplessness scale scores. Arthritis Care Res 1996;9:463–72.
21. Callahan LF, Pincus T, Huston JW III, et al. Measures of activity and damage in rheumatoid arthritis: Depiction of changes and prediction of mortality over five years. Arthritis Care Res 1997;10:381–94.
22. Söderlin MK, Nieminen P, Hakala M. Functional status predicts mortality in a community based rheumatoid arthritis population. J Rheumatol 1998;25:1895–9.
23. Sokka T, Hakkinen A, Krishnan E, et al. Similar prediction of mortality by the health assessment questionnaire in patients with rheumatoid arthritis and the general population. Ann Rheum Dis 2004;63:494–7.
24. Sokka T, Abelson B, Pincus T. Mortality in rheumatoid arthritis: 2008 update. Clin Exp Rheumatol 2008;26:S35–61.
25. Pincus T, Wolfe F. An infrastructure of patient questionnaires at each rheumatology visit: improving efficiency and documenting care. J Rheumatol 2000;27:2727–30.
26. Pincus T, Yazici Y, Bergman M. Development of a multidimensional health assessment questionnaire (MDHAQ) for the infrastructure of standard clinical care. Clin Exp Rheumatol 2005;23:S19–28.
27. Fries JF, Spitz P, Kraines RG, et al. Measurement of patient outcome in arthritis. Arthritis Rheum 1980;23:137–45.
28. Pincus T, Summey JA, Soraci SA Jr, et al. Assessment of patient satisfaction in activities of daily living using a modified Stanford health assessment questionnaire. Arthritis Rheum 1983;26:1346–53.

29. Wolfe F, Michaud K, Pincus T. Development and validation of the health assessment questionnaire II: a revised version of the health assessment questionnaire. Arthritis Rheum 2004;50:3296–305.
30. Pincus T, Swearingen C, Wolfe F. Toward a multidimensional health assessment questionnaire (MDHAQ): assessment of advanced activities of daily living and psychological status in the patient friendly health assessment questionnaire format. Arthritis Rheum 1999;42:2220–30.
31. Pincus T, Sokka T, Kautiainen H. Further development of a physical function scale on a multidimensional health assessment questionnaire for standard care of patients with rheumatic diseases. J Rheumatol 2005;32:1432–9.
32. Ware JE Jr, Sherbourne CD. The MOS 36-item short-form health survey (SF-36): I. Conceptual framework and item selection. Med Care 1992;30:473–81.
33. Ware J Jr, Kosinski M, Keller SD. A 12-item short-form health survey: construction of scales and preliminary tests of reliability and validity. Med Care 1996;34:220–33.
34. Fries JF, Ramey DR. Arthritis-specific global health analog scales assess generic health-related quality-of-life in patients with rheumatoid arthritis. J Rheumatol 1997;24:1697–702.
35. van der Heijde DM, van't Hof M, van Riel PL, et al. Development of a disease activity score based on judgment in clinical practice by rheumatologists. J Rheumatol 1993;20:579–81.
36. Hurst NP, Jobanputra P, Hunter M, et al. Validity of Euroqol—a generic health status instrument—in patients with rheumatoid arthritis. Br J Rheumatol 1994; 33:655–62.
37. Melzack R. The short-form McGill Pain Questionnaire. Pain 1987;30:191–7.
38. Krupp LB, LaRocca NG, Muir-Nash J, et al. The fatigue severity scale: application to patients with multiple sclerosis and systemic lupus erythematosus. Arch Neurol 1989;46:1121–3.
39. Tugwell P, Bombardier C, Buchanan WW, et al. The MACTAR patient preference disability questionnaire - an individualized functional priority approach for assessing improvement in physical disability in clinical trials in rheumatoid arthritis. J Rheumatol 1987;14:446–51.
40. Clinch J, Tugwell P, Wells G, et al. Individualized functional priority approach to the assessment of health related quality of life in rheumatology. J Rheumatol 2001;28:445–51.
41. Bellamy N, Buchanan WW, Goldsmith CH, et al. Validation study of WOMAC: a health status instrument for measuring clinically important patient relevant outcomes to antirheumatic drug therapy in patients with osteoarthritis of the hip or knee. J Rheumatol 1988;15:1833–40.
42. Burckhardt CS, Clark SR, Bennett RM. The fibromyalgia impact questionnaire: development and validation. J Rheumatol 1991;18:728–33.
43. Fries JF, Bruce B, Cella D. The promise of PROMIS: using item response theory to improve assessment of patient-reported outcomes. Clin Exp Rheumatol 2005;23: S53–7.
44. Hewlett S, Kirwan J, Pollock J, et al. Patient initiated outpatient follow up in rheumatoid arthritis: six-year randomised controlled trial. Br Med J 2005;330:171–4.
45. Pincus T, Gibofsky A, Weinblatt ME. Urgent care and tight control of rheumatoid arthritis as in diabetes and hypertension: better treatments but a shortage of rheumatologists. Arthritis Rheum 2002;46:851–4.
46. Wolfe F, Pincus T, Thompson AK, et al. The assessment of rheumatoid arthritis and the acceptability of self-report questionnaires in clinical practice. Arthritis Care Res 2003;49:59–63.

47. Russak SM, Croft JD, Furst DE, et al. The use of rheumatoid arthritis health-related quality of life patient questionnaires in clinical practice: lessons learned. Arthritis Care Res 2003;49:574–84.
48. Aletaha D, Smolen J, Ward MM. Measuring function in rheumatoid arthritis: identifying reversible and irreversible components. Arthritis Rheum 2006;54: 2784–92.
49. Yazici Y, Kautiainen H, Sokka T. Differences in clinical status measures in different ethnic/racial groups with early rheumatoid arthritis: implications for interpretation of clinical trial data. J Rheumatol 2007;34:311–5.
50. Pincus T, Callahan LF. Rheumatology function tests: grip strength, walking time, button test and questionnaires document and predict long-term morbidity and mortality in rheumatoid arthritis. J Rheumatol 1992;19:1051–7.
51. Pincus T. Rheumatology function tests: quantitative physical measures to monitor morbidity and predict mortality in patients with rheumatic diseases. Clin Exp Rheumatol 2005;23:S85–9.
52. Pincus T, Brooks RH, Callahan LF. Reliability of grip strength, walking time and button test performed according to a standard protocol. J Rheumatol 1991;18: 997–1000.

The Disease Activity Score and the EULAR Response Criteria

Jaap Fransen, PhD*, Piet L.C.M. van Riel, MD, PhD

KEYWORDS

- Rheumatoid arthritis • Disease Activity Score
- EULAR • Response criteria

The Disease Activity Score (DAS), its modified version the DAS28, and the DAS-based European League Against Rheumatism (EULAR) response criteria are well-known measures of disease activity in rheumatoid arthritis (RA). The DAS and the DAS28 consist of a combination of the number of tender joints, the number of swollen joints, erythrocyte sedimentation rate (ESR), and a global assessment rating by the patient.[1–3] The EULAR response criteria are calculated with the DAS or the DAS28 using the individual change in disease activity and the level of disease activity reached to classify trial participants as good, moderate, or nonresponders.[4–7]

The DAS, DAS28, and the EULAR response criteria have been extensively validated.[8] Their use in RA clinical trials and for monitoring patients who have RA is still increasing. The DAS28 is included in the American College of Rheumatology 2008 Recommendations for the Use of Nonbiologic and Biologic Disease-Modifying Antirheumatic Drugs in Rheumatoid Arthritis as an outcome measure on which to base treatment decisions.[9] The DAS and DAS28 were used in several clinical trials that showed the beneficial effects of tight control for the treatment of RA.[10–12] For applying tight control principles in practice, and for interpreting results from clinical trials, the DAS used in RA are relevant for clinicians to know.

This article updates previous summaries[8,13] on the development and validation of the DAS, DAS28, and EULAR response criteria and their use in research and clinical practice.

THE DISEASE ACTIVITY SCORE

The DAS was originally developed as an index containing the Ritchie Articular Index (RAI, range, 0–78), a 44 swollen joint count (range, 0–44), ESR, and a patient global

A version of this article originally appeared in the 21:4 issue of *Best Practice & Research: Clinical Rheumatology*.

Department of Rheumatology, Radboud University Nijmegen Medical Centre, P.O. Box 9101, NL-6500HB Nijmegen, The Netherlands

* Corresponding author.

E-mail address: J.Fransen@reuma.umcn.nl (J. Fransen).

Rheum Dis Clin N Am 35 (2009) 745–757
doi:10.1016/j.rdc.2009.10.001
0889-857X/09/$ – see front matter © 2009 Elsevier Inc. All rights reserved.

assessment on a visual analog scale (range, 0–100).[2,3] A specially programmed DAS calculator and a computer program that can be downloaded from the Internet are available to calculate the DAS (**Table 1**). The DAS has a continuous scale ranging from 0 to 10, and usually shows a Gaussian distribution in populations that have RA (**Fig. 1**). The level of disease activity can be interpreted as low (DAS ≤2.4), moderate (2.4<DAS ≤3.7), or high (DAS>3.7).[5] A DAS less than 1.6 corresponds with being in remission according to the American Rheumatism Association (ARA) criteria.[14] The DAS is reasonably well related to patient global assessment of disease activity (**Fig. 2**), despite the little weight that the patient-assessed global item received in the DAS formula. Therefore, the DAS also reflects patient-assessed disease activity.

Development of the Disease Activity Score

The DAS was developed using a large prospective study, in which decisions of rheumatologists to initiate or discontinue disease-modifying antirheumatic drug (DMARDs) treatment because of disease remission were equated with high and low disease activity, respectively.[1,2] High disease activity was characterized as either start of a DMARD or termination of DMARD treatment because of lack of effect. Low disease activity was characterized as either termination of DMARD treatment because of RA remission, not changing a DMARD for at least 1 year, or not starting DMARD treatment for at least 1 year. To develop the DAS, various statistical methods were used to identify the clinical and laboratory variables that explained most of the variation in rheumatologists' decisions on DMARD treatment, according to factor analysis, defining disease activity, discriminant analysis, regression analysis, and reproducibility.

Factor Analysis

A factor analysis was performed on the individual data, resulting in a five-factor model. The factors could be labeled as shown in **Box 1**.

Defining Disease Activity

The rheumatologists' decisions on initiating and terminating DMARDs were used as an external standard to define high and low disease activity. The clinical assessments were performed by specially trained research nurses, and the rheumatologists made all decisions concerning DMARDs independently of these assessments. The rheumatologists were not aware that their decisions were part of the investigation.

Discriminant Analysis

The factor values of the five factors were entered into a discriminant analysis, using assessments during defined high and low disease activity. Factors 3 and 5 were

---

Table 1
Computation of the disease activity score

Disease activity score (four variables) =
  DAS–4 = 0.53938*√(Ritchie) + 0.06465*(swollen joints) + 0.330*ln(ESR) + 0.00722*(GH)

Disease activity score (three variables) =
  DAS–3 = 0.53938*√(Ritchie) + 0.06465*(swollen joints) + 0.330*ln(ESR) + 0.224

Abbreviations: DAS, Disease Activity Score; ESR, erythrocyte sedimentation rate; GH, general health; Ritchie, Ritchie articular index; swollen joints, 44 swollen joint count.
Data from Van der Heijde DMFM, Van 't Hof MA, Van Riel PLCM, et al. Development of a Disease Activity Score based on judgment in clinical practice by rheumatologists. J Rheumatol 1993;20: 579–81.

The DAS was developed using DMARD decisions on real RA patients as external standard of low and high disease activity.

- The DAS uses only **4 selected items**, to avoid double-counting of information
- The DAS uses **weights**, for the same reason
- The DAS uses the √ and ln **transformations** to provide a Gaussian distribution.

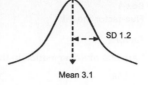

Ritchie=Ritchie Articular Index, Swollen joints=44 Swollen Joint Count, ESR=Erythrocyte Sedimentation Rate (Westergren), GH=General Health (100mm. VAS)

Fig. 1. Anatomy of the Disease Activity Score (DAS).

omitted, because grip strength also reflects destruction, and protein analysis has low reproducibility. No discriminating power was lost by omitting these factors.

Regression Analysis

A stepwise forward multiple regression analysis was used to determine which variables explained the greatest part of the discriminant function, with ESR, hemoglobulin, thrombocytes, morning stiffness, number of tender joints, number of swollen joints, Ritchie score, pain, patient global assessment, CRP, and IgM-RF as independent 2variables. Based on these results, the DAS was composed using the Ritchie score, number of swollen joints, ESR, and patient global assessment (see **Table 1**).

Reproducibility

The reproducibility of the DAS was determined by an interperiod correlation matrix of repeated measurements over 5 months. The measurement–remeasurement correlation was 0.89 for the DAS with three and four variables.

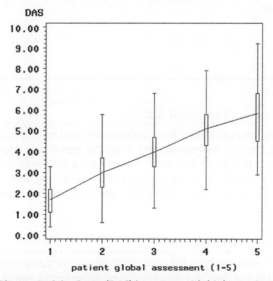

Fig. 2. The mean Disease Activity Score (DAS) increases with higher ratings on a 1 to 5 Likert scale for patient-assessed global disease activity in patients who have rheumatoid arthritis from a clinical trial. (*From* Van Ede AE, Laan RF, Rood MJ, et al. Effect of folic or folinic acid supplementation on the toxicity and efficacy of methotrexate in rheumatoid arthritis: a forty-eight week, multicenter, randomized, double-blind, placebo-controlled study. Arthritis Rheum 2001;44(7):1515–24; with permission.)

Box 1
Five-factor model

Factor 1

Variables of inflammation in the blood

    ESR

    Thrombocytes

    Hemoglobulin

    C-reactive protein (CRP)

    Rheumatoid factor of IgM (IgM-RF)

Factor 2

Variables of the joint examination

    Ritchie score

    Tender joints

    Swollen joints

Factor 3

Protein analysis

    Albumin and α-, β-, and γ-globulins

Factor 4

Subjective complaints

    Pain

    General health

    Morning stiffness

Factor 5

Impairment

    Grip strength

In Early and Established Rheumatoid Arthritis

The DAS was developed using data from patients who had recent-onset (<3 years) RA. Later, a new DAS formula was developed using the same procedure and the same cohort, with up to 9 years of follow-up.[3] The resulting DAS was almost identical to the DAS as developed in the early-onset sample, indicating that disease duration did not influence the construction of the DAS and was not necessary to replace the original DAS.

Validity of the Disease Activity Score

The DAS includes measures from the core set of measures that are used to assess the efficacy of DMARDs, but the DAS deliberately excludes measures of disability or joint damage.[1,2] The DAS showed greater power than other indices or single variables to discriminate low from high disease activity as defined by DMARD changes,[15] and also showed a good capacity to discriminate active RA from partial or complete remission in another study.[16] Furthermore, the DAS had the highest correlations with single measures and other composite indices, used to estimate disease activity,[15,17] indicating that the combination of several variables into an index was advantageous. The DAS also correlated significantly with disability as measured with the Health Assessment Questionnaire (HAQ),[15,18] and an increase in the DAS was associated with an increase in disability over the same period.[19] Also, the value of the DAS over time was well related to the amount of increase in joint damage over the same period (**Fig. 3**).[15,20] One study also showed that fluctuations in DAS scores contribute to progression of joint damage.[20]

DEVELOPMENT AND VALIDITY OF THE DISEASE ACTIVITY SCORE (DAS28)

The DAS28 is an index similar to the original DAS, consisting of a 28 tender joint count (range, 0–28), a 28 swollen joint count (range, 0–28), ESR, and facultatively, a patient global assessment on a visual analog scale (range, 0–100) (**Table 2**).[3] Because of the use of reduced and nongraded joint counts, the DAS28 is easier to complete than the DAS. The DAS28 has a continuous scale ranging from 0 to 9.4, and usually shows a Gaussian distribution in RA populations. DAS and DAS28 values cannot be directly compared, but a formula to transform DAS28 into DAS values is available.[6] The level of disease activity can be interpreted as low (DAS28 $\leq$ 3.2), moderate (3.2<DAS28 $\leq$ 5.1), or high (DAS28>5.1).[6]

A DAS less than 2.6 corresponds with being in remission according to the ARA criteria,[21] meaning that nearly all patients in remission have a DAS28 less than 2.6; however, not all patients who have a DAS28 less than 2.6 are in remission. A change of 1.2 (two times the measurement error) of the DAS28 in an individual patient is considered a significant change.[6] The EULAR response criteria can also be applied using the DAS28.[6]

The development of the DAS28 mirrored the development of the DAS.[3] The same cohort was used, but with more patients included and a longer duration of follow-up. It was concluded that no capacity to discriminate between low and high disease activity was lost by replacing the two comprehensive joint counts by the

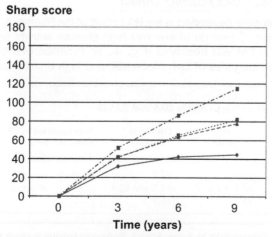

Fig. 3. Progression of joint damage is dependent on having a constant low Disease Activity Score (DAS) (*lower curve*), a fluctuating low or constant high DAS (*middle curves*), or a fluctuating high DAS (*upper curve*). (*From* Welsing PMJ, Landewe, RB, Van Riel PLCM, et al. The relationship between disease activity and radiologic progression in patients with rheumatoid arthritis: a longitudinal analysis. Arthritis Rheum 2004;50(7):2082–93; with permission.)

Table 2
Computation of the modified disease activity scores using 28 joint counts

Modified disease activity score (four variables) =
   DAS28–4 = 0.56*√(TJC28) + 0.28*√(SJC28) + 0.70*ln(ESR) + 0.014*(General Health)

Modified disease activity score (three variables) =
   DAS28–3 = [0.56*√(TJC28) + 0.28*√(SJC28) + 0.70*ln(ESR)]1.08 + 0.16

Abbreviations: DAS, Disease Activity Score; ESR, erythrocyte sedimentation rate; GH, general health; SJC28, 28 swollen joint count; TJC28, 28 tender joint count.

Data from Prevoo MLL, Van 't Hof MA, Kuper HH, et al. Modified disease activity scores that include twenty-eight-joint counts. Development and validation in a prospective longitudinal study of patients with rheumatoid arthritis. Arthritis Rheum 1995;38(1):44–8.

28 joint count. The correlation of the modified DAS (DAS28) with the original DAS was 0.97.

The DAS28 was validated using data from the same cohort and data from a similar cohort.[3] Similar correlations of the DAS and DAS28 with the Mallya index, HAQ, and grip strength were found, with no differences between the cohorts. The correlations of the DAS and DAS28 with radiographically visible joint damage were also similar.

DEVELOPMENT AND VALIDITY OF THE EULAR RESPONSE CRITERIA

The EULAR response criteria incorporate the amount of change, and a certain level of disease activity,[7,22] much like the newly developed ACR hybrid response criteria.[23] The EULAR response criteria classify patients as good, moderate, or nonresponders, using the individual amount of change in DAS and the level (low, moderate, or high) of DAS reached (**Table 3**).[5] A change of 1.2 (two times the measurement error of 0.6) of the DAS in an individual patient is considered a significant change.[5] For example, a patient must show a significant change ($\Delta DAS > -1.2$), but must also reach low disease activity (DAS ≤ 2.4) to be classified as a good responder. The EULAR response criteria can also be applied using the DAS28 (see **Table 3**).[6]

Development of the EULAR Response Criteria

The EULAR criteria were developed in the RA cohort of the Radboud University Nijmegen Medical Center.[5,6] Periods of low and high disease activity were also defined using decisions on DMARD treatment (**Fig. 4**). To minimize overlap, the DAS was divided into three categories of low, moderate, and high disease activity. To define

Table 3
The EULAR response criteria using the DAS and DAS28

Disease Activity Level	DAS at Endpoint	DAS28 at Endpoint	Improvement in DAS or DAS28 From Baseline		
			>1.2	>0.6 and ≤1.2	≤0.6
"low"	≤2.4	≤3.2	good		
"moderate"	>2.4 and ≤3.7	>3.2 and ≤5.1		moderate	
"high"	>3.7	>5.1			none

Abbreviations: DAS, Disease Activity Score; EULAR, European League Against Rheumatism.

Data from Van Gestel AM, Prevoo MLL, Van 't Hof MA, et al. Development and validation of the European League Against Rheumatism response criteria for rheumatoid arthritis. Arthritis Rheum 1996;39(1):34–40 and Van Gestel AM, Haagsma CJ, Van Riel PLCM. Validation of rheumatoid arthritis improvement criteria that include simplified joint counts. Arthritis Rheum 1998;41(10):1845–50.

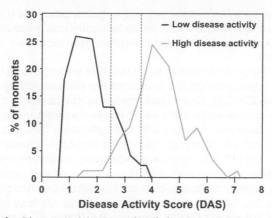

Fig. 4. Borders in the Disease Activity Score (DAS) discriminating low, moderate, and high disease activity. (*From* Van Gestel AM, Prevoo MLL, Van 't Hof MA, et al. Development and validation of the European League Against Rheumatism response criteria for rheumatoid arthritis. Arthritis Rheum 1996;39(1):34–40; with permission.)

relevant change, the measurement error of the DAS was estimated using linear regression of the interperiod correlations through estimating the measurement–remeasurement correlation r_0 (correlation between DAS measurements with intermediate time interval of 0). From r_0 the measurement error was calculated as 0.6.

Validity of the EULAR Response Criteria

The resulting EULAR response criteria (see **Table 3**) were validated in several clinical trials.[5–7] The ACR improvement criteria and EULAR response criteria agreed reasonably well. Patients who were good or moderate responders showed significantly more improvement in functional capacity and less progression of joint damage than those who experienced no response.[7]

The validity of the EULAR criteria was confirmed in a study analyzing nine well-performed clinical trials that covered a range and differences in response between treatment groups.[7] The investigators concluded that ACR and EULAR definitions of response in RA performed similarly in discriminating active or experimental treatment from placebo or control treatment. In addition, the ACR and EULAR definitions of response performed comparably in association with overall assessments of improvement and progression of joint damage.

USE OF THE DISEASE ACTIVITY SCORE AND EULAR CRITERIA IN CLINICAL TRIALS

Although the ACR improvement criteria and the DAS-based EULAR response criteria use a different approach, both perform well in distinguishing placebo from active treatment and in discriminating between two types of active treatment.[7,24] The DAS-based EULAR response criteria were developed to compare treatments in clinical trials, but the DAS can also be used for this purpose as a continuous end point; then, the difference between two drugs or drug and placebo can readily be interpreted in terms of the DAS. The advantage of using a continuous DAS is that no loss of power occurs from categorization. Also, when no success or failure cut point is used, more precision is available to assess the benefits of effective treatments. Especially when response criteria are relatively easy to fulfill, the effectiveness of the treatment may be underestimated. However, when response criteria are too difficult to fulfill, none of the patients in the treatment arms may be responders and an actual difference between two treatments cannot be shown. However, cut points for continuous measures may be useful as (secondary) trial end points when the categories have prognostic meaning and are clinically meaningful.

When using the DAS, cut points may be chosen that are dependent on the trial objectives. An example is using the DAS28 to indicate low disease activity (DAS28 ≤ 3.2) or near-remission (DAS28<2.6). One reason for using cut points is that measures of success or failure are generally more easily interpreted than continuous measures. Interpretation of a response measure with two categories (yes and no), as with the ACR improvement criteria, is simpler than for a response measure that has three categories, as with the EULAR response criteria (good, moderate, and none).

The number of patients who have a DAS28 less than 2.6 (near-remission) is a much-used secondary outcome measure in clinical trials, which also has practical meaning. However, because the DAS28 is an average, some patients may have two or more swollen joints and still have a DAS28 less than 2.6 (**Table 4**). A stricter definition is the Outcome Measures in Rheumatoid Arthritis Clinical Trials (OMERACT) definition of *minimal disease activity* that can be calculated using the DAS28 (**Fig. 5**).[25]

In the next decade, more effective treatment for RA will become available, and measures such as time-to-remission or time-spent-in-remission may become useful as end points in clinical trials. These end points can already be measured using the DAS and DAS28, and more strict cut points may be chosen when appropriate.

USING THE DISEASE ACTIVITY SCORE IN CLINICAL PRACTICE

For clinical practice, experts generally agree that rheumatoid inflammation should be controlled as soon as possible and as completely as possible, and that control should be maintained for as long as possible, consistent with patient safety.[26] With the goal of treatment to attain and sustain low disease activity or even remission, the management of RA should clearly include systematic and regular quantitative evaluation of rheumatoid inflammation.[27] These principles are now widely known as *tight control* in the treatment of RA.[28]

Table 4
Examples of different disease activity parameters and the resulting DAS28

28 TJC	28 SJC	ESR	GH	DAS28	Level
0	0	20	10	2.24	low
1	0	20	10	2.80	low
1	1	20	10	3.08	low
2	0	20	50	3.50	moderate
2	2	30	50	4.27	moderate
4	0	30	50	4.20	moderate
4	4	30	50	4.76	moderate
8	0	50	70	5.30	high
8	8	50	70	6.09	high

The scores were calculated according to the formula in **Table 2**. The level of disease activity can be interpreted as low (DAS28 ≤ 3.2), moderate (3.2<DAS28 ≤ 5.1), or high (DAS28>5.1).
Abbreviations: DAS, Disease Activity Score; ESR, erythrocyte sedimentation rate; GH, general health; SJC, swollen joint count; TJC, tender joint count.

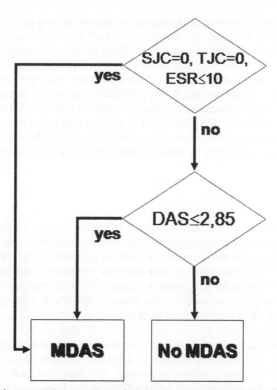

Fig. 5. An algorithm to arrive at minimal disease activity (MDA) using the DAS28. DAS, Disease Activity Score; ESR, erythrocyte sedimentation rate; MDAS, minimal disease activity state; SJC, swollen joint count; TJC, tender joint count. (*From* Wells GA, Boers M, Shea B, et al. Minimal disease activity for rheumatoid arthritis: a preliminary definition. J Rheumatol 2005;32(10):2016–24; with permission.)

For the assessment of rheumatoid inflammation in daily clinical practice, it is advantageous that the DAS and DAS28 are measures used in clinical studies, especially clinical trials. This use facilitates knowledge transfer, or evidence-based practice, because study results are easier to transfer to one's own practice. Furthermore, because the DAS and DAS28 are measures with absolute value, they are suitable for determining and evaluating the status and course of disease activity in patients who have RA. Relative measures, such as the ACR improvement criteria, cannot be used for that purpose.[27] However, interpretation of an index may be difficult in practice, but is facilitated when more experience and more (predictive) knowledge are available. Some examples of DAS28 values at different levels of clinical disease activity are given in **Table 4**.

In practice, the DAS28 may seem to be more feasible than the DAS because of the reduced and nongraded joint counts. However, although the DAS and DAS28 can support clinical decision making, they do not replace careful patient examination and inquiry. Nonetheless, systematic monitoring of inflammatory activity may serve several goals in practice, such as for recognizing whether the therapy chosen is necessary and effective, ensuring that rheumatoid inflammation remains under control, and adjusting DMARD therapy.[26–28]

Monitoring alone has no benefit on health, but an appropriate treatment may. Perhaps the best example of this is the Tight Control of Rheumatoid Arthritis (TICORA) study, in which DMARD therapy was steadily increased as long as the DAS was higher than 2.4 (a DAS ≤ 2.4 is called *low disease activity*).[10] Patients treated intensively had a greater mean decrease in DAS, were more likely to be in remission (65% vs. 16%), had more reduction of disability, and experienced less progression of joint damage[10] compared with those treated with a usual care strategy. In a comparable monitoring trial [Tracking Rheumatoid Arthritis Activity (TRAC)], the choice of treatment strategy was freely determined by the clinician, whereas only the guideline to reach low disease activity according to the DAS28 (DAS28 ≤ 3.2) was applied in the intervention group.[11] However, the effect in the TRAC trial was much less than the effect in the TICORA trial, which may be explained largely by the lower intensity of the treatment that was used in the TRAC study.

DISCUSSION

RA is a multifaceted disorder, and therefore measurement of multiple outcomes is relevant to its management, including disease activity, disability, and joint damage.[29] The core-set of outcome measures to be used in RA clinical trials of DMARDs illustrates this, including a measure for joint damage, a measure for disability, and six measures to reflect the underlying disease activity.[29] The complexity of finding a single representative outcome measure for RA disease activity is related to that of the pathogenic process and multiple joint involvement.

Currently, no gold standard measure exists for RA disease activity. Imaging techniques, such as MRI and ultrasound, and biomarkers are promising objective disease activity measures, especially at subclinical levels of disease activity.[30–32] However, their relevance for clinical practice is unclear. For daily practice, patient-reported outcomes, such as the RADAI, HAQ, or RAPID, have the advantage that no laboratory values and no formal joint counts are required.[33–37] However, many rheumatologists may be hesitant to omit a joint count or ESR, which are still seen as important sources of information.

To increase validity and precision, RA disease activity measures have long been combined in a pooled measure to increase validity and precision.[38] A famous first example is the Lansbury index, which contained ESR, morning stiffness, fatigue, pain, and grip strength.[38] The DAS and DAS28 consist of a combination of the number of tender joints, the number of swollen joints, ESR, and a global assessment rating by the patient.[3,4] If no global rating is available, it may also be omitted. Instead of ESR, the DAS can also be calculated using CRP (www.das-score.nl). Consequently, several formulas are available for calculating the DAS and DAS28, respectively, which may cause some confusion.[39] Values of the DAS and DAS28 are not directly comparable, but a transformation formula is available. The simplified disease activity index (SDAI) and clinical disease activity index (CDAI) are derivations of the DAS28 that add a physician global estimate and omit the weighting (SDAI) and a laboratory value (CDAI).[40]

The DAS and DAS28 have several advantages: (1) they reflect the extent of underlying inflammation, unlike a change measure such as ACR20, (2) they reflect a clinical meaningful target of antirheumatic treatment (low disease activity), (3) because of the incorporation of a measure with absolute value (DAS or DAS28), responses to treatments in clinical trials can be compared meaningfully, especially also in comparative/nonsuperiority trials, (4) they will also be useful in future trials of highly effective DMARDs, and (5) trial results can be expressed in a clinically meaningful outcome that can be translated into clinical use.

The main disadvantages of indices such as the DAS include concerns over validity and practical problems, such as interpretation and computational difficulties.[38] The validity of an index depends on that of the measures that are included and their appropriate weighting. The interpretation of an index becomes easier when more information (eg, discriminative or predictive) from validity studies is available and when familiarity with an index is increasing.

Meanwhile, the DAS, DAS28, and EULAR response criteria have been extensively validated and are increasingly used in RA clinical trials and to monitor patients who have RA.[8,27] However, although the DAS is a useful guide for treatment decisions, it does not replace careful patient examination and inquiry. Self-assessment of RA disease activity may be less laborious for the physician than assessing the DAS, and may ensure physicians have included the patient perspective on disease activity. Patient assessment of disease activity is reasonably well related to the DAS but is not sufficiently identical to replace the DAS by with patient-reported outcomes.[33]

Several clinical trials have shown that a tight control strategy, including measurement of disease activity, target setting, and planned adjustment of antirheumatic medication, is an effective treatment for RA.[10–12] With awareness of these results, patients and clinicians should be ready to apply outcome measurement in their practices. The DAS and DAS28 are valid measures and have been shown to be suitable measures to apply in a tight control strategy for treating RA.

REFERENCES

1. Van der Heijde DMFM, Van 't Hof MA, Van Riel PLCM, et al. Judging disease activity in clinical practice in rheumatoid arthritis: first step in the development of a Disease Activity Score. Ann Rheum Dis 1990;49:916–20.
2. Van der Heijde DMFM, Van 't Hof MA, Van Riel PLCM, et al. Development of a Disease Activity Score based on judgment in clinical practice by rheumatologists. J Rheumatol 1993;20:579–81.
3. Prevoo MLL, Van 't Hof MA, Kuper HH, et al. Modified Disease Activity Scores that include twenty-eight-joint counts. Development and validation in a prospective longitudinal study of patients with Rheumatoid Arthritis. Arthritis Rheum 1995; 38(1):44–8.
4. Riel van PLCM, Gestel van AM, Putte van de LBA. Development and validation of response criteria in rheumatoid arthritis: steps towards an international consensus on prognostic markers. Br J Rheumatol 1996;35(Suppl 2):4–7.
5. Van Gestel AM, Prevoo MLL, Van 't Hof MA, et al. Development and validation of the European league against rheumatism response criteria for rheumatoid arthritis. Arthritis Rheum 1996;39(1):34–40.
6. Van Gestel AM, Haagsma CJ, Van Riel PLCM. Validation of rheumatoid arthritis improvement criteria that include simplified joint counts. Arthritis Rheum 1998; 41(10):1845–50.
7. Van Gestel AM, Anderson JJ, Van Riel PLCM, et al. ACR and EULAR improvement criteria have comparable validity in rheumatoid arthritis trials. J Rheumatol 1999; 26:705–11.
8. Fransen J, Stucki G, Van Riel PLCM. Rheumatoid arthritis measures. Arthritis Rheum 2003;49(5S):S214–24.
9. Saag KG, Teng G G, Patkar NM, et al. American college of rheumatology 2008 recommendations for the use of nonbiologic and biologic disease-modifying antirheumatic drugs in rheumatoid arthritis. Arthritis Rheum 2008; 59(6):762–84.

10. Grigor C, Capell HA, Stirling A, et al. Effect of a treatment strategy of tight control for rheumatoid arthritis (the TICORA study): a single-blind randomised controlled trial. Lancet 2004;364:263–9.
11. Fransen J, Moens BH, Speyer I, et al. The effectiveness of systematic monitoring of RA disease activity in daily practice (TRAC): a multi centre, cluster-randomised controlled trial. Ann Rheum Dis 2005;64(9):1294–8.
12. Goekoop-Ruiterman YP, de Vries-Bouwstra JK, Kerstens PJ, et al. DAS-driven therapy versus routine care in patients with recent-onset active Rheumatoid Arthritis. Ann Rheum Dis 2009, Jan 20. [Epub ahead of print].
13. Fransen J, van Riel PLCM. The Disease Activity Score and the EULAR response criteria. Clin Exp Rheumatol 2005;23(Suppl 39):S93–9.
14. Prevoo MLL, Van Gestel AM, Van 't Hof MA, et al. Remission in a prospective study of patients with rheumatoid arthritis. Br J Rheumatol 1996;35:1101–5.
15. Van der Heijde DMFM, Van 't Hof MA, Van Riel PLCM, et al. Validity of single variables and composite indices for measuring disease activity in rheumatoid arthritis. Ann Rheum Dis 1992;51:177–81.
16. Salaffi F, Peroni M, Ferraccioli GF. Discriminating ability of composite indices for measuring disease activity in rheumatoid arthritis: a comparison of the chronic arthritis systemic index, Disease Activity Score and Thompson's articular index. Rheumatology 2000;39:90–6.
17. Villaverde V, Balsa A, Cantalejo M, et al. Activity indices in rheumatoid arthritis. J Rheumatol 2000;27(11):2576–81.
18. Drossaers-Bakker KW, De Buck M, Van Zeben D, et al. Long-term course and outcome of functional capacity in rheumatoid arthritis. Arthritis Rheum 1999; 42(9):1854–60.
19. Welsing PMJ, Van Gestel AM, Swinkels HL, et al. The relationship between disease activity, joint destruction, and functional capacity over the course of rheumatoid arthritis. Arthritis Rheum 2001;44(9):2009–17.
20. Welsing PMJ, Landewe RB, Van Riel PLCM, et al. The relationship between disease activity and radiologic progression in patients with rheumatoid arthritis: a longitudinal analysis. Arthritis Rheum 2004;50(7):2082–93.
21. Fransen J, Creemers MCW, Van Riel PLCM. Remission in rheumatoid arthritis: agreement of the Disease Activity Score (DAS28) with the ARA preliminary remission criteria. Rheumatology 2004;43(10):1252–5.
22. Van Riel PL, Reekers P, Van de Putte LB, et al. Association of HLA antigens, toxic reactions and therapeutic response to auranofin and aurothioglucose in patients with rheumatoid arthritis. Tissue Antigens 1983;22(3):194–9.
23. American College of Rheumatology Committee to Reevaluate Improvement Criteria. A proposed revision to the ACR20: the hybrid measure of American college of rheumatology. Arthritis Rheum 2007;57(2):193–202.
24. Verhoeven AC, Boers M, Van der Linden S. Responsiveness of the core set, response criteria, and utilities in early rheumatoid arthritis. Ann Rheum Dis 2000;39:966–74.
25. Wells GA, Boers M, Shea B, et al. Minimal disease activity for rheumatoid arthritis: a preliminary definition. J Rheumatol 2005;32(10):2016–24.
26. Wolfe F, Cush JJ, O'Dell JR, et al. Consensus recommendations for the assessment and treatment of rheumatoid arthritis. J Rheumatol 2001;28:1413–30.
27. Fransen J, Stucki G, Van Riel PLCM. The merits of monitoring: should we follow all our rheumatoid arthritis patients in daily practice? Rheumatology (Oxford) 2002; 41:601–4.

28. Kiely PDW, Brown AK, Edwards CJ, et al. Contemporary treatment principles for early rheumatoid arthritis: a consensus statement. Rheumatology (Oxford) 2009; 48(7):765–72.
29. Felson DT, Anderson JJ, Boers M, et al. The American college of rheumatology preliminary core-set of disease activity measures for rheumatoid arthritis clinical trials. Arthritis Rheum 1993;36(6):729–40.
30. Farrant JM, O'Connor PJ, Grainger AJ. Advanced imaging in rheumatoid arthritis. Part 1: synovitis. Skeletal Radiol 2007;36(4):269–79.
31. Farrant JM, Grainger AJ, O'Connor PJ. Advanced imaging in rheumatoid arthritis: part 2: erosions. Skeletal Radiol 2007;36(5):381–9.
32. Emery P, Gabay C, Kraan M, et al. Evidence-based review of biologic markers as indicators of disease progression and remission in rheumatoid arthritis. Rheumatol Int 2007;27(9):793–806.
33. Fransen J, Langenegger T, Michel BA, et al. Feasibility and validity of the RADAI, a self-administered rheumatoid arthritis disease activity index. Rheumatology (Oxford) 2000;39:321–7.
34. Pincus T, Swearingen CJ, Bergman M, et al. RAPID3 (routine assessment of patient index data 3), a rheumatoid arthritis index without formal joint counts for routine care: proposed severity categories compared to DAS and CDAI categories. J Rheumatol 2008;35:2136–47.
35. Pincus T, Bergman MJ, Yazici Y, et al. An index of only patient-reported outcome measures, routine assessment of patient index data 3 (RAPID3), in two abatacept clinical trials: similar results to Disease Activity Score (DAS28) and other RAPID indices that include physician-reported measures. Rheumatology (Oxford) 2008;47(3):345–9.
36. Wolfe F, Michaud K, Pincus T. A composite disease activity scale for clinical practice, observational studies, and clinical trials: the patient activity scale (PAS/PAS-II). J Rheumatol 2005;32(12):2410–5.
37. Bruce B, Fries JF. The health assessment questionnaire (HAQ). Clin Exp Rheumatol 2005;23(5 Suppl 39):S14–8.
38. Boers M, Tugwell P. The validity of pooled outcome measures (indices) in rheumatoid arthritis clinical trials. J Rheumatol 1993;20:568–74.
39. Van der Heijde DMFM, Jacobs JWG. The original DAS and the DAS28 are not interchangeable: comment on the articles by Prevoo et al. Arthritis Rheum 1998;41(5):942–3 Van Riel PLCM, Van Gestel AM. Reply. Arthritis Rheum 1998;41(5):943–5.
40. Aletaha D, Smolen J. The simplified disease activity index (SDAI) and the clinical disease activity index (CDAI): a review of their usefulness and validity in rheumatoid arthritis. Clin Exp Rheumatol 2005;23(5 Suppl 39):S100–8.

The Simplified Disease Activity Index and Clinical Disease Activity Index to Monitor Patients in Standard Clinical Care

Daniel Aletaha, MD, MS*, Josef S. Smolen, MD

KEYWORDS

- Clinical disease activity index • Simplified disease activity index
- Disease activity score 28 • Rheumatoid arthritis

THE TRIAD AND INTERRELATIONSHIP OF DISEASE ACTIVITY, JOINT DAMAGE, AND FUNCTIONAL IMPAIRMENT

Synovitis is the cardinal consequence of the pathogenetic events of inflammatory joint diseases. The type of synovitis encountered by patients with rheumatoid arthritis (RA) contrasts that of other arthritides by its high propensity to destroy bone and cartilage. Although the causes of RA remain enigmatic, some light has been shed on the mechanisms leading to the disease, which comprise, among other events, overexpression of proinflammatory cytokines.[1,2] Surrogates of inflammation include the acute-phase response and the degree of clinical disease activity, the major expressions of which are pain, stiffness, and swelling of the joints.[3–5] However, the degree of disease activity is also closely related to the extent of joint destruction.[6–8]

Yet another characteristic of RA is the severe functional impairment that can occur early in its course and that constitutes the sequel of the disease that is most important to the patients. The serious corollaries of RA physical disability are a reduction of quality of life,[9] rapid loss of working capacity,[10] and premature mortality.[9,11] Although

A version of this article originally appeared in the 21:4 issue of *Best Practice & Research: Clinical Rheumatology*.

Division of Rheumatology, Department of Internal Medicine III, Medical University of Vienna, Waehringer Guertel 18-20, A-1090 Vienna, Austria

* Corresponding author.

E-mail address: daniel.aletaha@meduniwien.ac.at (D. Aletaha).

physical disability is caused primarily by joint pain and stiffness, it is also a result of joint damage.[12–14] Although functional impairment caused by inflammatory pain is fully reversible, the accrual of joint damage over the course of time leads to an increase of the irreversible fraction of disability. This irreversibility can be assessed in states of clinical remission when reversible components related to disease activity are absent and cannot influence disability.[12] Thus, the inflammatory processes leading to synovitis are linked with the processes directing cartilage and bone damage and the combined effects of activity and joint damage steer disability (**Fig. 1**). Even though the inflammatory and the destructive response can be disentangled under certain circumstances,[15] this linkage between inflammation/disease activity, destruction, and disability is a principal, a fundamental, association in the disease: the "triad" of RA.

THE CENTRAL ROLE OF DISEASE ACTIVITY AND ITS EVALUATION

The central role of disease activity in the triad is based on its direct causation of disability and its elicitation of joint damage, which indirectly leads to functional impairment. Thus, control of disease activity is the pivotal therapeutic goal in RA. This has clearly been shown in many studies, including trials on the effects of various therapies,

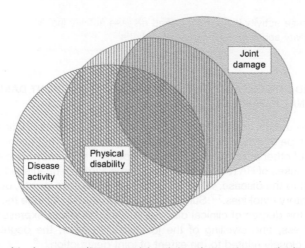

Fig. 1. Relationship between disease activity, joint destruction, and physical disability. Disease activity (*thick hatching*) is the major cause of disability (*thin vertical hatching*) and joint damage (*gray*). Very mild or subclinical disease activity might not be afflicted with disability or damage (*thickly lined only*). In some patients, disease activity is high enough to cause functional impairment, but joint destruction might not occur (*overlay of thick and thin lines*), and, progression of joint damage, even in patients with active disease, is often seen in less than 50% of patients with RA; in these individuals disability is fully reversible. In another group, there is high disease activity, functional impairment, and destruction (*overlay of all 3 shades*), and disability is only partially reversible. Some patients are in a remission-like state, might have experienced little joint damage, and consequently might not suffer from significant reduction in physical function (*gray only*). There is also a group of patients who are in remission but have had severe destruction in the past and consequently suffer from irreversible functional impairment (*overlay of gray and thin hatching*). There might also be RA patients who have no residual disease activity and have not experienced major cartilage and bone destruction but have damage to periarticular structures or muscle weakness resulting in some degree of physical disability (*thin vertical hatching*).

such as biologic agents,[16–22] and investigations aiming at analyzing management strategies.[23,24] More reduction in disease activity is associated with better radiographic and functional outcomes[16–20] and patients whose therapy was switched when they were not reaching a predetermined category of low disease activity, as assessed by composite indices, fare much better than those followed by traditional questioning and nonstructured ways of changing therapy.[23,24]

THE OBSTACLES TO FOLLOWING DISEASE ACTIVITY

Controlling disease activity by evaluating its clinical and laboratory characteristics has been a challenge in rheumatology. Reliable evaluation has been possible for about a decade, using the RA core set variables[25–27] and response criteria or indices that reflect improvement on therapeutic intervention or actual disease activity.[28–30] However, it is still not easy to motivate rheumatologists to use such methods in routine practice, and even distributing questionnaires on physical function, which is one element of the core set, to patients seems difficult in daily practice.[31]

Given that no cardiologist would neglect to examine the heart or measure blood pressure and that no neurologist would neglect performing a neurologic examination, it is surprising that rheumatologists are often satisfied with not assessing the organs involved in disorders such as RA, namely the joints. Time constraints, however, must be acknowledged, and any examination methods used should be as simple as possible. Moreover, in an ideal world, the physician and the patient would speak a similar, if not the same, language, so that the same information can be shared among those involved with RA and those caring for them.

TRADITIONAL INSTRUMENTS TO EVALUATE DISEASE ACTIVITY AND ITS IMPROVEMENT

Over the decades, numerous scores or response criteria have been developed to evaluate disease activity at a single time point or (absolute or relative) improvement of disease activity.[32] In the 1990s, the American College of Rheumatology (ACR) developed response criteria[28] based on the improvement of the ACR core data set variables. These criteria were designed to differentiate between active treatment and placebo in clinical trials. The criteria have limitations in clinical practice because they require a reference measurement (in clinical trials, this would be the baseline measurement), because of their dichotomous nature (ie, providing a yes/no answer about a level of improvement), and because of their inability to provide results on a continuous scale reflecting actual disease activity. This last limitation was partially addressed when the numerical ACR response was introduced (ACR-N),[33] although this also contains some inadequacies.[34,35] Importantly, however, the ACR response criteria were a major step forward because they relied on changes of a group of variables rather than on individual signs and symptoms of RA, in line with the notion that composite indices would mirror RA disease activity more effectively than individual variables.[5,36]

A pivotal step forward in disease activity assessment was the development of the Disease Activity Score (DAS) by a group in Nijmegen.[29,37] This constitutes a composite score based on tender and swollen joint counts and patient assessment of global health and erythrocyte sedimentation rate (ESR). For the first time, this score allowed a reliable evaluation of disease activity on a continuous scale, of changes of actual disease activity in the course of therapy, and of response evaluation based on these changes.[38] Determining a value of the DAS required extended joint examinations for swelling and grading joints for tenderness by the Ritchie index. A nomogram, or calculator, was also necessary because of the complex nature of the formula (**Table 1**), which had been derived by statistical optimization algorithms. Although the transformation of the original DAS to the DAS-28, which uses a 28-joint count, was successfully achieved[30] to enable the use of reduced joint counts while obviating grading tender joints, the complexity of the formula and the necessity to use a calculator or computer program did not change (see **Table 1**).

SIMPLIFIED DISEASE ACTIVITY INDEX AND CLINICAL DISEASE ACTIVITY INDEX

After nearly a decade, a new generation of scores has been developed, in line with current insights about the importance of close monitoring of patients and the value of active involvement of patients in the process of controlling disease activity in other fields of medicine.[39,40] Major limitations with the earlier scoring systems were the complexity of the then-available indices, such as those based on the DAS, which were obstacles to effective patient involvement and consequential clinical use (no calculator, no DAS). These limitations resulted in questions as to whether the complexity of the DAS and DAS-28 was truly necessary for reliable assessment of disease activity or whether the scoring method could further be simplified. Research in reactive arthritis outcome measurement indicated that a straightforward scoring method, which required only the numerical summation of 5 of the traditional core set variables, was perfectly reliable in the assessment of disease activity. This score was called the Disease Activity Index for Reactive Arthritis (DAREA),[41] and the transposition of the thinking behind the DAREA to RA led to the development of the Simplified Disease Activity Index (SDAI, see **Table 1**). The SDAI revealed a surprisingly good correlation with the DAS-28.[42] The correlation of the SDAI with functional impairment as evaluated by the Health Assessment Questionnaire (HAQ) or with radiographic progression was very similar to that of the DAS-28, and the correlation with the HAQ remained virtually unchanged when C-reactive protein (CRP) was eliminated from the formula, which then contained only the 2 joint counts and the 2 global assessments.[42]

This further simplified score (see **Table 1**), which used only clinically accessible variables and was therefore named Clinical Disease Activity Index (CDAI), was also validated and proved to correlate well not only with the DAS-28, the ACR response, and the HAQ, but also, over time, with radiographic changes to a virtually identical degree as the DAS-28 and the SDAI.[7] The latter analyses revealed that the

Table 1
Disease activity indices: calculation and cutpoints of disease activity categories

Index	Formula	Cutpoints
DAS-28	$0.56 \times \sqrt{(TJC28)} + 0.28 \times \sqrt{(SJC28)} + 0.70 \times \text{lognat(ESR)} + 0.014 \times GH$	<2.6/<3.2/<5.1[a]
SDAI	SJC28 + TJC28 + PGA + EGA + CRP	≤3.3/≤11/≤26
CDAI	SJC28 + TJC28 + PGA + EGA	≤2.8/≤10/≤22

Abbreviations: CDAI, Clinical Disease Activity Index; CRP, C-reactive protein; DAS-28, DAS based on a 28-joint count; EGA, evaluator global assessment of disease activity; GH, global health; PGA, patient global assessment of disease activity; SDAI, Simplified Disease Activity Index; SJC, swollen joint count; TJC, tender joint count.
[a] Remission vs low disease activity/low vs moderate disease activity/moderate vs high disease activity GH in mm Visual Analog Scale (VAS); SDAI: CRP in mg/dl; SDAI, CDAI: PGA, EGA in cm on a VAS.

acute-phase response did not provide essential information beyond the 2 joint counts and global assessments when incorporated in the composite index. Importantly, the CDAI allowed the assessment of disease activity without the need to wait for laboratory results. Although there are other ways to overcome this problem (such as instructing patients to obtain laboratory results separately from the clinical visit) or to calculate indices at a later point in time (when the results have been received), the CDAI allowed more effective disease activity assessment and particularly warranted the possibility of immediate treatment decisions on the spot for all patients all the time.

Furthermore, the information conveyed by the acute-phase reactants can still be obtained and interpreted independently. Although there is generally a high correlation between clinical variables and the acute-phase response, it is advantageous to exclude the acute-phase response from a disease activity formula because, in clinical practice, the clinical assessment would typically overrule the information provided by acute-phase response levels. For example, if very high CRP levels are clearly not related to a relatively mild clinical disease activity, the clinician will search for other reasons for the elevation of CRP levels, such as an infection, rather than considering the disease to be more active. Likewise, a disproportionately low CRP level or ESR would probably not affect disease activity considerations in patients with high clinical disease activity, if at all. In this scenario, the acute-phase response could potentially modify the choice of treatment but not influence the necessity of a change in treatment. In addition, Wolfe and Michaud[43] observed that about 40% of patients with RA have normal ESR or CRP level at presentation and that some patients do not have a change in their ESR and CRP level despite clinical change.[44] Therefore, the inclusion of the acute-phase reactant not only complicates clinical assessment because of its frequent unavailability but also might actually detract from the capacity to monitor patients optimally. For all these reasons, it can be argued that the acute-phase response should be part of disease activity evaluation (as considered in the core sets) but is not necessarily needed as an integral part of disease activity indices.

The SDAI and the CDAI have been validated in many studies and shown to perform well when compared with other indices across different cultures.[45–51] Moreover, physician decisions to modify disease-modifying antirheumatic drug (DMARD) therapy correlate better with changes of SDAI and CDAI than with changes in other instruments.[48,49] The fact that changes in SDAI and CDAI correlate highly with changes of the HAQ in the course of clinical trials and that these 3 scores are linear rather than mathematically transformed allowed the calculation of the component of the HAQ that is related to disease activity (ACT-HAQ). This HAQ/SDAI value is higher in early RA than in established RA. The attribution of a value to the ACT-HAQ ultimately enabled deriving the component of the HAQ that is related to joint damage (DAM-HAQ), which was found to be relatively constant irrespective of disease duration.[52]

Disease Activity States by SDAI and CDAI

Disease activity categories have been defined for both the SDAI and the CDAI (see **Table 1**). These categories are correlated significantly with those of the DAS-28,[45,46] except for the category of remission, in which SDAI and CDAI are more stringent.[45,46,53–55] However, remission appears to be the optimal state to be aimed for when treating RA for several reasons. First, patients with long-term remission by SDAI or CDAI have no or little radiographic progression of joint damage when compared with those with moderate and high disease activity.[4,56] Second, there appear to be fewer radiographic changes in remission than in even a state of low disease activity.[4] Third, in patients with short disease duration or little radiographic damage, functional disability is fully reversible when states of remission by SDAI (or

CDAI) are achieved.[47] And fourth, when the stringent definition of remission, as by SDAI or CDAI, is used in the longer term, the residual disability might be lower than that of remission according to the DAS-28 criteria,[4,55,57] probably because of the higher residual joint counts that are frequently observed in DAS-28 remission.[45,54] **Fig. 2** shows 3 scenarios of very low disease activity or, as it would be judged by most rheumatologists,[4] remissions that lead to identical SDAI and CDAI but discrepant DAS-28 values.

Current treatment strategies allow remission to be achieved in a significant proportion of patients. This proportion might be exaggerated if the DAS-28 criteria are used,[16,20,58] but stringent sustained remission by SDAI and CDAI can be observed in 17% to 18% of patients in clinical practice.[55] Further, on the individual patient level, the stringency of SDAI and CDAI remission is revealed by the fact that with increasing duration of remission there is a vast decrease in the proportion of patients who show any radiologic progression.[59]

Response Criteria for SDAI and CDAI

In the context of therapy, it is also important to find out how a patient responds to a given treatment approach. To this end, preliminary response criteria have been developed for the SDAI and the CDAI to better judge the proportions of patients responding.[60] Clearly, the categories of low disease activity or, better, remission are the desired therapeutic states. However, given that even in states of high disease activity the degree of baseline activity is somewhat predictive of future structural outcome,[61] major improvement, even if not leading to a more desired disease state, might not only provide information on the effect of a given therapeutic modality but also reduce overall disease activity, with likely new prospects for subsequent therapies. From a patient perspective, when looking at patient satisfaction with therapy,

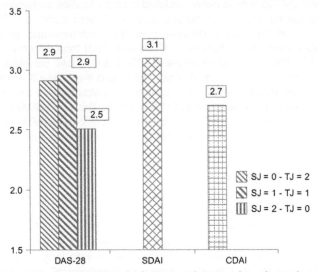

Fig. 2. Three case representations in which SDAI and CDAI values showed consistent remission and DAS-28 changed between remission and low disease activity. In all these cases, the joint counts (swollen and/or tender joints) equaled 2, patient global assessment was 4 mm (0.4 cm), evaluator global assessment was 3 mm (0.3 cm), ESR ¼ was 19 mm, and CRP ¼ was 0.4 mg/dL.

the change in SDAI or CDAI needs to be greater with higher disease activity, again providing evidence that the attainment of a particular state is more important than a particular change in disease activity.[62]

Application of SDAI and CDAI in Clinical Practice

The therapeutic approach in the authors' clinics is based on a modification of a recently published algorithm,[63] which was validated by real-life, tightly controlled studies of patients with RA whose therapy was adjusted accordingly.[23,24] To comply with this algorithm (**Fig. 3**) and to allow for immediate decision making without needing to wait for any laboratory results, the CDAI is applied, which can be determined from joint counts and global assessments (see **Table 1**) and which does not require CRP level or ESR. Thus, at every visit, the physician determines the CDAI, the value of which is communicated to the patients ('Know your CDAI!'). These visits, in the very early phases of DMARD therapy, are spaced about 6 weeks apart, and subsequently, depending on the degree of disease activity, every 3 to 6 months.

Whereas in states of moderate or high disease activity (CDAI>10) determining the CDAI alone is usually sufficient to draw conclusions about change of therapy, in the low disease activity range (CDAI≤10) it is important to judge the composition of the index: if the patient global assessment is dominant and joint counts are very low, the result might be because of coexisting fibromyalgia, depression, or similar conditions. This would also be a problem if ACR response criteria or the DAS-28 was used. Under these circumstances, antirheumatic therapy would not need to be altered. However, if a CDAI within the low disease activity state was driven primarily by swollen joint counts, therapeutic modification would be considered. ESR or CRP levels can provide additional information in situations of low disease activity, as discussed earlier.

The authors use the CAre for RA database (CARAbase), which they developed several years ago, to follow the patients thoroughly. **Fig. 4** depicts 3 typical follow-up curves of CDAI and SDAI for patients with (1) immediate excellent response, (2) protracted good response after several DMARD changes, and (3) improvement but resistance to reaching low disease activity or remission.

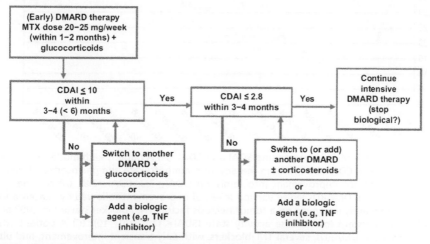

Fig. 3. Algorithm for optimizing therapy by tight control using the CDAI. MTX, methotrexate; TNF, tumor necrosis factor. (*Data from* Aletaha D, Smolen JS, Kvien TK. Definition of moderate and major response for disease activity indices in rheumatoid arthritis. Ann Rheum Dis 2006;65(Suppl II):692.)

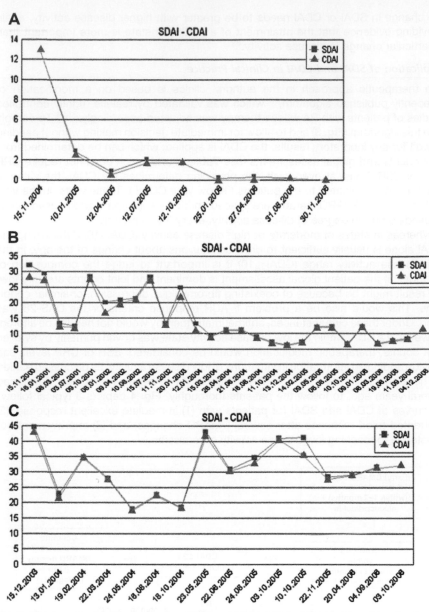

Fig. 4. Three patient follow-ups using SDAI and CDAI. (*A*) A patient with moderate disease activity (SDAI>11, CDAI>10) in whom therapy with methotrexate and glucocorticoids led to rapid and sustained improvement into remission (SDAI≤3.3, CDAI≤2.8). (*B*) A patient in whom traditional DMARDs led to varying levels of improvement followed by exacerbation and who ultimately improved on a tumor necrosis factor (TNF) blocker started in 2003 and reached a consistent low disease activity state (SDAI≤11, CDAI≤10). (*C*) A patient who received various DMARDs, several TNF blockers, with only transient improvement, and ultimately rituximab (October 2006) without ever reaching even a moderate disease activity state (SDAI≤26, CDAI≤22). Note that in the last visits only CDAIs were recorded, as CRP level was missing and SDAI could not be calculated. Dates read as DD/MM/YYYY. (*Courtesy of* Department of Internal Medicine III, Medical University of Vienna, Austria, copyright; with permission. Copyright © 2009.)

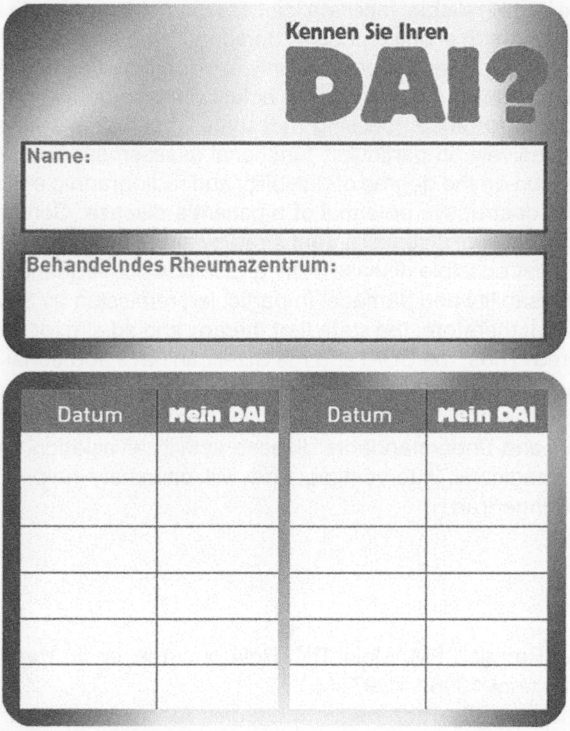

Fig. 5. Credit-card-sized patient diary for entering CDAI values with every visit. (*Top*) Front page: Do you know your DAI? Name of patient, name of rheumatologic center. (*Bottom*) Back page: date, my DAI. (*Courtesy of* Department of Internal Medicine III, Medical University of Vienna, Austria, copyright; with permission. Copyright © 2009.)

All the patients receive a credit-card-sized CDAI diary (**Fig. 5**) that allows them to enter their actual CDAI at every outpatient visit and thus to monitor their disease activity. In this way, they are fully informed and reminded to request actual information on their disease activity status at every visit. Likewise, given the simple numerical summation used to determine the CDAI, increments in the CDAI have clinical correlates (eg, "one more joint affected" or "1 cm more on a global scale"). Well-informed patients tend to be more compliant with therapy, with consequently better long-term outcomes. In the same way, the consistency in disease activity assessment achieved by composite indices also improves outcomes, and the CDAI allows direct implementation of newer strategies, such as tight control[24,63] in clinical and nonclinical settings.

SUMMARY

Evaluation of disease activity in RA is not trivial. No single marker can reflect all aspects of the disease. Disease activity instruments, such as scores, criteria, and indices, have significantly improved the rheumatologist's ability to evaluate the course of RA. All that is required is the performance of formal joint counts, which is not an unreasonable requirement for physicians dealing with joint diseases. Reduced joint counts, which are highly reliable, facilitate joint assessment even more and can be performed easily by nonmedical office or clinic personnel who have received the required (brief) training. However, the authors not only advocate the use of instruments that reflect the disease process and inform on actual disease activity, its changes, and its state but also call for encompassing measures of outcome to evaluate patients' disease comprehensively. In particular, functional assessment by the HAQ provides important information on the degree of disability and radiographic evaluation provides information on the destructive potential of a patient's disease. Conversely, using the SDAI or the CDAI as part of an assessment strategy and adapting therapy accordingly to achieve the lowest possible disease activity also has consequences in the prevention of long-term disability and damage. In particular, remission by SDAI/CDAI criteria is very stringent and, therefore, the state that therapy should aim for before tapering of drugs is considered. Thus, the CDAI and the SDAI can have additional advantages, as they advance the disease activity instrument to incorporate a second role, which is potentially even more significant. This role derives from the collateral effects of consistent, consequent, and understandable disease activity evaluation, which in itself is a strategic, not medicinal, intervention, and will ultimately help improve disease outcomes in the longer run.

REFERENCES

1. Feldmann M, Brennan FM, Maini RN. Role of cytokines in rheumatoid arthritis. Annu Rev Immunol 1996;14:397–440.
2. Smolen JS, Steiner G. Therapeutic strategies for rheumatoid arthritis. Nat Rev Drug Discov 2003;2:473–88.
3. Mallya RK, de Beer FC, Hamilton ED, et al. Correlation of clinical parameters of disease activity in rheumatoid arthritis with serum concentrations of C-reactive protein and erythrocyte sedimentation rate. J Rheumatol 1982;9:224–8.
4. Aletaha D, Machold KP, Nell VPK, et al. The perception of rheumatoid arthritis core set measures by rheumatologists. Results of a survey. Rheumatology 2006;45:1133–9 [Epub Mar 7, 2006].
5. van der Heijde DM, Van't Hof MA, van Riel PL, et al. Validity of single variables and composite indices for measuring disease activity in rheumatoid arthritis. Ann Rheum Dis 1992;51:177–81.
6. van Leeuwen MA, van Rijswijk MH, Sluiter WJ, et al. Individual relationship between progression of radiological damage and the acute phase response in early rheumatoid arthritis. Towards development of a decision support system. J Rheumatol 1997;24(1):20–7.
7. Aletaha D, Nell VPK, Stamm T, et al. Acute phase reactants add little to composite disease activity indices for rheumatoid arthritis: validation of a clinical activity score. Arthritis Res 2005;7:R796–806.
8. van Leeuwen MA, Van der Heijde DM, van Rijswijk MH, et al. Interrelationship of outcome measures and process variables in early rheumatoid arthritis. A comparison of radiologic damage, physical disability, joint counts, and acute phase reactants. J Rheumatol 1994;21(3):425–9.
9. Pincus T, Callahan LF, Sale WG, et al. Severe functional declines, work disability, and increased mortality in seventy-five rheumatoid arthritis patients studied over nine years. Arthritis Rheum 1984;27:864–72.
10. Sokka T, Kautiainen H, Mottonen T, et al. Work disability in rheumatoid arthritis 10 years after the diagnosis. J Rheumatol 1999;26(8):1681–5.

11. Pincus T, Callahan LF. Early mortality in RA predicted by poor clinical status. Bull Rheum Dis 1992;41(4):1–4.
12. Aletaha D, Smolen JS, Ward MM. Measuring function in rheumatoid arthritis: identifying reversible and irreversible components. Arthritis Rheum 2006;54: 2784–92.
13. Drossaers-Bakker KW, de Buck M, van Zeben D, et al. Long-term course and outcome of functional capacity in rheumatoid arthritis: the effect of disease activity and radiologic damage over time. Arthritis Rheum 1999;42:1854–60.
14. Welsing PM, van Gestel AM, Swinkels HL, et al. The relationship between disease activity, joint destruction, and functional capacity over the course of rheumatoid arthritis. Arthritis Rheum 2001;44(9):2009–17.
15. Smolen JS, Han C, Bala M, et al. Evidence of radiographic benefit of infliximab plus methotrexate in rheumatoid arthritis patients who had no clinical improvement: a detailed subanalysis of the ATTRACT trial. Arthritis Rheum 2005;52: 1020–30.
16. Breedveld FC, Weisman MH, Kavanaugh AF, et al. The PREMIER study - A multi-center, randomized, double-blind clinical trial of combination therapy with adali-mumab plus methotrexate versus methotrexate alone or adalimumab alone in patients with early, aggressive rheumatoid arthritis who had not had previous methotrexate treatment. Arthritis Rheum 2006;54:26–37.
17. Keystone EC, Kavanaugh AF, Sharp JT, et al. Radiographic, clinical, and functional outcomes of treatment with adalimumab (a human anti-tumor necrosis factor monoclonal antibody) in patients with active rheumatoid arthritis receiving concomitant methotrexate therapy: a randomized, placebo-controlled, 52-week trial. Arthritis Rheum 2004;50:1400–11.
18. Klareskog L, van der Heijde D, de Jager JP, et al. Therapeutic effect of the combination of etanercept and methotrexate compared with each treatment alone in patients with rheumatoid arthritis: double-blind randomised controlled trial. Lancet 2004;363:675–81.
19. Lipsky PE, Van der Heijde DM, St Clair EW, et al. Infliximab and methotrexate in the treatment of rheumatoid arthritis. Anti-Tumor Necrosis Factor Trial in Rheumatoid Arthritis with Concomitant Therapy Study Group. N Engl J Med 2000;343(22): 1594–602.
20. St Clair EW, van der Heijde DM, Smolen JS, et al. Combination of infliximab and methotrexate therapy for early rheumatoid arthritis: a randomized controlled trial. Arthritis Rheum 2004;50:3432–43.
21. Cohen S, Emery P, Greenwald M, et al. Rituximab for rheumatoid arthritis refractory to anti-tumor necrosis factor therapy. Arthritis Rheum 2006;54:2739–806.
22. Kremer JM, Genant HK, Moreland LW, et al. Effects of abatacept in patients with methotrexate-resistant active rheumatoid arthritis: a randomized trial. Ann Intern Med 2006;144(12):865–76.
23. Goekoop-Ruiterman YP, de Vrie-Bouwstra JK, Allaart CF, et al. Clinical and radiographic outcomes of four different treatment strategies in patients with early rheumatoid arthritis (the BeSt study): a randomized, controlled trial. Arthritis Rheum 2005;52:3381–90.
24. Grigor C, Capell H, Stirling A, et al. Effect of a treatment strategy of tight control for rheumatoid arthritis (the TICORA study): a single-blind randomised controlled trial. Lancet 2004;364:263–9.
25. Boers M, Tugwell P, Felson DT, et al. WHO and ILAR core endpoints for symptom modifying antirheumatic drugs in RA clinical trials. J Rheumatol 1994;21(Suppl 41):86–9.

26. Felson DT, Anderson JJ, Boers M, et al. The American College of Rheumatology preliminary core set of disease activity measures for rheumatoid arthritis clinical trials. Arthritis Rheum 1993;36:729–40.

27. Scott DL, Panayi GS, van Riel PL, et al. Disease activity in rheumatoid arthritis-preliminary report of the Consensus Study Group of the European workshop for rheumatology research. Clin Exp Rheumatol 1992;10:521–5.

28. Felson DT, Anderson JJ, Boers M, et al. American College of Rheumatology preliminary definition of improvement in rheumatoid arthritis. Arthritis Rheum 1995;38:727–35.

29. Van der Heijde DM, van't Hof M, van Riel PL, et al. Development of a disease activity score based on judgement in clinical practice by rheumatologists. J Rheumatol 1993;20:579–81.

30. van Gestel AM, Haagsma CJ, van Riel PL. Validation of rheumatoid arthritis improvement criteria that include simplified joint counts. Arthritis Rheum 1998; 41:1845–50.

31. Pincus T, Wolfe F. An infrastructure of patient questionnaires at each rheumatology visit: improving efficiency and documenting care [editorial]. J Rheumatol 2000;27:2727–30.

32. Aletaha D, Smolen JS. The definition and measurement of disease modification in inflammatory rheumatic diseases. Rheum Dis Clin North Am 2006;32:9–44.

33. Siegel JN, Zhen BG. Use of the American College of Rheumatology N (ACR-N) index of improvement in rheumatoid arthritis. Argument in favor. Arthritis Rheum 2005;52:1637–41.

34. Boers M. Use of the American College of Rheumatology N (ACR-N) index of improvement in rheumatoid arthritis. Argument in opposition. Arthritis Rheum 2005;52:1642–5.

35. Aletaha D, Smolen JS. The American College of Rheumatology N (ACR-N) debate: going back into the middle of the tunnel? Comment on the articles by Siegel and Zhen and by Boers. Arthritis Rheum 2006;54(1):377–8.

36. Goldsmith CH, Boers M, Bombardier C, et al. Criteria for clinically important changes in outcomes: development, scoring and evaluation of rheumatoid arthritis patients and trial profiles. J Rheumatol 1993;20:561–5.

37. van der Heijde DM, van't Hof MA, van Riel PL, et al. Judging disease activity in clinical practice in rheumatoid arthritis: first step in the development of a disease activity score. Ann Rheum Dis 1990;49:916–20.

38. van Gestel AM, Prevoo ML, van't Hof MA, et al. Development and validation of the European League Against Rheumatism response criteria for rheumatoid arthritis. Comparison with the preliminary American College of Rheumatology and the World Health Organization/International League Against Rheumatism Criteria. Arthritis Rheum 1996;39:34–40.

39. Egan BM, Lackland DT, Cutler NE. Awareness, knowledge, and attitudes of older Americans about high blood pressure: implications for health care policy, education, and research. Arch Intern Med 2003;163(6):681–7.

40. Rachmani R, Slavacheski I, Berla M, et al. Treatment of high-risk patients with diabetes: motivation and teaching intervention: a randomized, prospective 8-year follow-up study. J Am Soc Nephrol 2005;16(Suppl 1):S22–6.

41. Eberl G, Studnicka-Benke A, Hitzelhammer J, et al. Development of a disease activity index for the assessment of reactive arthritis (DAREA). Rheumatology 2000;39:148–55.

42. Smolen JS, Breedveld FC, Schiff MH, et al. A simplified disease activity index for rheumatoid arthritis for use in clinical practice. Rheumatology 2003;42:244–57.

43. Wolfe F, Michaud K. The clinical and research significance of the erythrocyte sedimentation rate. J Rheumatol 1994;21(7):1227–37.
44. Wolfe F, Pincus T. The level of inflammation in rheumatoid arthritis is determined early and remains stable over the longterm course of the illness. J Rheumatol 2001;28(8):1817–24.
45. Aletaha D, Ward MM, Machold KP, et al. Remission and active disease in rheumatoid arthritis: defining criteria for disease activity states. Arthritis Rheum 2005;52:2625–36.
46. Aletaha D, Smolen J. The Simplified Disease Activity Index (SDAI) and the Clinical Disease Activity Index (CDAI): a review of their usefulness and validity in rheumatoid arthritis. Clin Exp Rheumatol 2005;23(Suppl 39):S100–8.
47. Aletaha D, Smolen J, Ward MM. Measuring function in rheumatoid arthritis: identifying reversible and irreversible components. Arthritis Rheum 2006;54(9):2784–92.
48. American College of Rheumatology Committee to Reevaluate Improvement Criteria. A proposed revision to the ACR20: the hybrid measure of American College of Rheumatology response. Arthritis Rheum 2007;57:193–202.
49. Soubrier M, Zerkak D, Gossec L, et al. Which variables best predict change in rheumatoid arthritis therapy in daily clinical practice? J Rheumatol 2006;33(7):1243–6.
50. Lissiane K, Guedes N, Kowalski SC, et al. The new indices SDAI and CDAI in early arthritis: similar performance to the DAS28 index. Arthritis Rheum 2006;54(Suppl):S206–7.
51. Lian TY, Koh ET, RA study group TTSH, et al. Clinical Disease Activity Index (CDAI) is a valid instrument for assessing disease activity amongst oriental early rheumatoid arthritis (ERA) patients. Arthritis Rheum 2006;54(Suppl):S377–8.
52. Smolen JS, Aletaha D, Grisar JC, et al. Estimation of a numerical value for joint damage-related physical disability in rheumatoid arthritis clinical trials. Ann Rheum Dis 2009 [Epub ahead of print].
53. Makinen H, Kautiainen H, Hannonen P, et al. Is DAS28 an appropriate tool to assess remission in rheumatoid arthritis? Ann Rheum Dis 2005;64:1410–3; DOI: 10.1136/ard.2005.037333. [originally published online 7 Jun 2005].
54. van der Heijde D, Klareskog L, Boers M, et al. Comparison of different definitions to classify remission and sustained remission: 1 year TEMPO results. Ann Rheum Dis 2005;64:1582–7.
55. Mierau M, Schoels M, Gonda G, et al. Assessing remission in clinical practice. Rheumatology 2007;46(6):975–9.
56. Molenaar ET, Voskuyl AE, Dijkmans BA. Functional disability in relation to radiological damage and disease activity in patients with rheumatoid arthritis in remission. J Rheumatol 2002;29(2):267–70.
57. Aletaha D, Smolen JS. Remission of rheumatoid arthritis: should we care about definitions? Clin Exp Rheumatol 2006;24(6 Suppl 43):S45–51.
58. Maini RN, Taylor PC, Szechinski J, et al. Double-blind randomized controlled clinical trial of the interleukin-6 receptor antagonist, tocilizumab, in European patients with rheumatoid arthritis who had an incomplete response to methotrexate. Arthritis Rheum 2006;54(9):2817–29.
59. Aletaha D, Funovits J, Breedveld FC, et al. Rheumatoid arthritis joint progression in sustained remission is determined by disease activity levels preceding the period of radiographic assessment. Arthritis Rheum 2009;60:1242–9.
60. Aletaha D, Smolen JS, Kvien TK. Definition of moderate and major response for disease activity indices in rheumatoid arthritis (RA). Ann Rheum Dis 2006;65(Suppl II):692.

61. Smolen JS, van der Heijde DM, St Clair EW, et al. Predictors of joint damage in patients with early rheumatoid arthritis treated with high-dose methotrexate without or with concomitant infliximab. Results from the ASPIRE trial. Arthritis Rheum 2006;54:702–10.

62. Aletaha D, Funovits J, Ward MM, et al. Perception of improvement in patients with rheumatoid arthritis varies with disease activity levels at baseline. Arthritis Rheum 2009;61(3):313–20.

63. Smolen JS, Sokka T, Pincus T, et al. A proposed treatment algorithm for rheumatoid arthritis: aggressive therapy, methotrexate, and quantitative measures. Clin Exp Rheumatol 2003;21(Suppl 31):S209–10.

RAPID3, an Index to Assess and Monitor Patients with Rheumatoid Arthritis, Without Formal Joint Counts: Similar Results to DAS28 and CDAI in Clinical Trials and Clinical Care

Theodore Pincus, MD[a],*, Yusuf Yazici, MD[a],
Martin J. Bergman, MD[b]

KEYWORDS

• RAPID3 (routine assessment of patient index data 3)
• DAS28 • CDAI • Rheumatoid arthritis (RA)

RAPID3 (routine assessment of patient index data 3) is an index that includes only the 3 patient-reported American College of Rheumatology (ACR) Core Data Set measures for rheumatoid arthritis (RA): physical function, pain, and patient global estimate of status.[1] Each of these individual measures is scored 0 to 10, for a total of 0 to 30. RAPID3 is included by the ACR among the indices used to measure RA disease activity,[2] along with the disease activity score 28 (DAS28),[3,4] simplified disease activity index (SDAI),[5] clinical disease activity index (CDAI),[5] rheumatoid arthritis disease

A version of this article originally appeared in the 21:4 issue of *Best Practice & Research: Clinical Rheumatology*.
[a] Division of Rheumatology, Department of Medicine, New York University School of Medicine and NYU Hospital for Joint Diseases, Room 1608, 301 East 17th Street, New York, NY 10003, USA
[b] Division of Rheumatology, Taylor Hospital, Ridley Park, PA, USA
* Corresponding author.
E-mail address: tedpincus@gmail.com (T. Pincus).

Rheum Dis Clin N Am 35 (2009) 773–778
doi:10.1016/j.rdc.2009.10.008
0889-857X/09/$ – see front matter © 2009 Elsevier Inc. All rights reserved.

activity index (RADAI),[6] and patient activity scale (PAS I/II).[7] All these indices give relatively similar information, as documented in this article.

RAPID3 can be calculated in 5 to 10 seconds, in contrast to 90 to 94 seconds for a formal 28-joint count, 106 seconds for a CDAI, and 114 seconds for a DAS28 (**Table 1**).[8,9] An index that requires less than 10% of the time of a CDAI or DAS28 appears attractive for use in usual care (as well as in clinical research). However, it is necessary to document that RAPID3 provides similar information to the DAS28 and CDAI. Evidence that RAPID3 meets these criteria and therefore might provide a quantitative guide to tight control of RA in usual clinical care, analogous to DAS28 and CDAI in clinical trials, is summarized in this article.

RAPID3 IS CORRELATED SIGNIFICANTLY WITH DAS28 AND CDAI IN CLINICAL TRIALS AND CLINICAL CARE

Comparisons of RAPID3 with DAS28 and CDAI in 285 patients seen in usual care indicated Spearman rank order correlation coefficients for DAS28 with RAPID3 of 0.66 (**Fig. 1**A), and for CDAI with RAPID3 of 0.74 (**Fig. 1**B), all highly significant ($P<.001$).[1] RAPID3 shares only 1 of 4 measures with DAS28 and CDAI (patient global estimate of status). Similar results have been found in data from clinical trials.[10]

The level of these correlation coefficients is considerably higher than the correlation coefficient in the database from which these correlations were observed of erythrocyte sedimentation rate (ESR) with C-reactive protein (CRP) of 0.51. ESR and CRP are regarded as measuring a similar construct of inflammation. Likewise, RAPID3 measures a construct of RA clinical status similar to DAS28 and CDAI.

RAPID3 DISTINGUISHES ACTIVE FROM CONTROL TREATMENTS AS EFFICIENTLY AS DAS28 IN CLINICAL TRIALS

The capacity of RAPID3 to distinguish active from control treatments has been documented to be similar to that of DAS28 and CDAI in clinical trials of methotrexate,[11] leflunomide,[11] adalimumab,[12] and abatacept.[10] For example, in the AIM (Abatacept in Inadequate responders to Methotrexate) trial, percentage improvement with abatacept compared with control treatment was 41.4% versus 21.0% according to DAS28, and 47.5% versus 23.4% according to RAPID3; differences between the treatment arms were 20.3% for DAS28 and 24.0% for RAPID3 (**Fig. 2**).[10] In the ATTAIN (Abatacept Trial in Treatment of Anti-TNF Inadequate Responders) trial, percentage improvement with abatacept compared with control treatment was 28.3% versus 9.4% according to DAS28, and 34.7% versus 9.9% according to RAPID3; differences between treatment arms were 19.0% for DAS28 and 24.9% for RAPID3 (see

Table 1	
Mean number of seconds to score selected RA measures and indices by 7 rheumatologists	
Measure/Index	**Mean Number of Seconds to Score**
28-joint count	90[8]/95[9]
HAQ-DI	42[8]
RAPID3 (0–10 scale)	9.6[8]/9.6[9]
RAPID3 (0–30 scale)	4.6[9]
CDAI	100.1[9]
DAS28	112.7[9]

Data from Refs.[8,9]

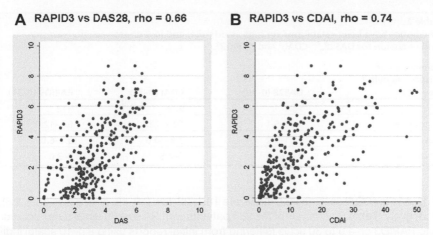

Fig. 1. Spearman rank order correlations of (*A*) RAPID3 versus DAS28 (ρ = 0.657) and (*B*) RAPID3 versus CDAI (ρ = 0.738) in 285 patients with rheumatoid arthritis. (*From* Pincus T, Swearingen CJ, Bergman M, et al. RAPID3 (routine assessment of patient index data 3), a rheumatoid arthritis index without formal joint counts for routine care: Proposed severity categories compared to DAS and CDAI categories. J Rheumatol 2008;35:2136–47; with permission.)

Fig. 1).[10] Therefore, RAPID3 distinguishes active from control treatments at levels similar to DAS28 in this trial, and to DAS28 as well as to CDAI in other clinical trials (presented at EULAR 2009—Annual European Congress of Rheumatology).

RAPID3 YIELDS SIMILAR CATEGORIES FOR HIGH, MODERATE, AND LOW ACTIVITY, AND REMISSION, COMPARED WITH DAS28 AND CDAI

Categories have been established for high, moderate, and low disease activity, and remission for DAS28 (ie, high >5.1, moderate 3.21–5.1, low 2.61–3.2, and remission

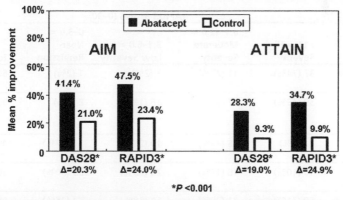

Fig. 2. Comparison of percentage change in DAS28 and RAPID3 scores in the AIM and ATTAIN clinical trials of abatacept in rheumatoid arthritis. (*Data from* Pincus T, Bergman MJ, Yazici Y, et al. An index of only patient-reported outcome measures, routine assessment of patient index data 3 (RAPID3), in 2 abatacept clinical trials: similar results to disease activity score (DAS28) and other RAPID indices that include physician-reported measures. Rheumatology (Oxford) 2008;47:345–9.)

Table 2
Categories have been established for high, moderate, and low disease activity/severity and remission for DAS28,[3,4] CDAI,[5] and RAPID3[1]

Categories of Disease Activity/ Severity	DAS28 (0–10)	CDAI (0–76)	RAPID3 (0–30)
High	>5.1	>22	>12
Moderate	3.21–5.1	10.1–22.0	6.1–12.0
Low	2.61–3.2	2.9–10.0	3.1–6.0
Remission	0–2.6	0–2.8	0–3.0

≤ 2.6), and for CDAI (ie, high >22, moderate 10.1–22, low 2.9–10, and remission ≤ 2.8), respectively (**Table 2**). Analysis of the 285 patients with RA seen in usual care[1] according to RAPID3 on a 0 to 30 scale (differing from initial reports using a 0–10 scale) indicated classification criteria of high severity greater than 12, moderate 6.1 to 12, low 3.1 to 6, and near-remission 3 or less.

Most patients who met criteria for each of these 4 disease severity categories according to RAPID3 scores were found to meet similar activity categories for DAS28 and CDAI (**Tables 3** and **4**). Overall, 81% to 84% of patients who met DAS28 or CDAI moderate-/high-activity criteria met similar RAPID3 severity criteria, and 68% to 70% who met DAS28 or CDAI low activity/remission criteria met similar RAPID3 criteria. Again, RAPID3 was as informative as indices that included a physician/assessor joint count or physician/assessor global estimate. Similar data have also been found in clinical trials[10] (presented at EULAR 2009).

As noted above, initial reports concerning RAPID3 described conversion of the 0 to 30 scale to a 0 to 10 scale.[1,10] However, scoring of RAPID3 on a 0 to 10 scale requires

Table 3
RAPID3 scores compared with DAS28 in 285 patients at 3 clinical rheumatology sites

	RAPID3 Scores (0–30)				
DAS28	>12 = High Severity	6.1–12.0 = Moderate Severity	3.1–6.0 = Low Severity	0–3.0 = Near- Remission	Total
>5.1 = high activity	37 (74%)	11 (22%)	1 (2%)	1 (2%)	50 (17%)
3.21–5.1 = moderate activity	39 (43%)	27 (30%)	16 (18%)	8 (9%)	90 (32%)
2.61–3.2 = low activity	4 (10%)	15 (38%)	10 (25%)	11 (27%)	40 (14%)
0–2.6 = remission	10 (10%)	18 (17%)	24 (23%)	53 (50%)	105 (37%)
Total	90 (31%)	71 (25%)	51 (18%)	73 (26%)	285

All percentages are row percentages, except total in rightmost column (column percentages). Kappa 0.26; weighted kappa 0.44.

Data from Pincus T, Swearingen CJ, Bergman M, et al. RAPID3 (routine assessment of patient index data 3), a rheumatoid arthritis index without formal joint counts for routine care: proposed severity categories compared to DAS and CDAI categories. J Rheumatol 2008;35:2136–47.

Table 4
RAPID3 scores compared with CDAI in 285 patients at 3 clinical rheumatology sites

CDAI	RAPID3 Scores (0–30)				
	>12 = High Severity	6.1–12.0 = Moderate Severity	3.1–6.0 = Low Severity	0–3.0 = Near-Remission	Total
>22 = High activity	39 (78%)	9 (18%)	1 (2%)	1 (2%)	50 (17%)
10.1–22.0 = Moderate activity	36 (40%)	33 (36%)	15 (17%)	6 (7%)	90 (32%)
2.9–10.0 = Low activity	15 (16%)	28 (30%)	25 (27%)	25 (27%)	93 (33%)
0–2.8 = Remission	0 (0%)	1 (2%)	10 (19%)	41 (79%)	52 (18%)
Total	90 (31%)	71 (25%)	51 (18%)	73 (26%)	285

All percentages are row percentages, except total in rightmost column (column percentages).
Kappa 0.32; weighted kappa 0.51.
Data from Pincus T, Swearingen CJ, Bergman M, et al. RAPID3 (routine assessment of patient index data 3), a rheumatoid arthritis index without formal joint counts for routine care: proposed severity categories compared to DAS and CDAI categories. J Rheumatol 2008;35:2136–47.

10 seconds, compared with only 5 seconds on a 0 to 30 scale, which is currently recommended.[9] The initial reports also described additional RAPID scores: RAPID4 added to RAPID3 a joint count, either a self-report RADAI joint count,[1,6] or standard 28 swollen and tender joint count.[10] RAPID5 added to RAPID4 a physician global estimate of status.[1,10] All RAPID indices were converted to a 0 to 10 scale through division by 3, 4, or 5 according to the number of measures included. Extensive analyses indicated that RAPID4 and RAPID5 yielded data similar to RAPID3 but required double the time for calculation on a 0 to 10 scale, 20 seconds instead of 10 seconds.[1,8,10] Therefore, RAPID3 on a 0 to 30 scale is recommended for use in usual care.

It should be emphasized that the authors do not advocate RAPID3 to replace indices that include joint counts and laboratory tests in clinical trials, and agree that the Core Data Set and DAS28 are preferred for their specificity.[13] Nonetheless, all Core Data Set measures had similar sensitivities to distinguish active from control treatments in multiple trials.[13] These observations support the validity of RAPID3 in usual clinical care.

Documentation of the similar sensitivity of RAPID3 to distinguish between active and control treatments in clinical trials should reassure clinicians that RAPID3 is informative in monitoring patients. In usual clinical care, the clinician is making decisions based not only on an index, but on a composite of findings from patient history, physical examination, laboratory tests, and imaging data. RAPID3 seems sufficient to document patient status in a quantitative manner, to compare from one visit to another, and to document a course over long periods.

The MDHAQ is easily completed by patients, and a RAPID3 score gives results that are similar to widely recognized indices, DAS28 and CDAI, but in 5 to 10 versus more than 100 seconds. Use of MDHAQ/RAPID3 by all rheumatologists could transform clinical rheumatology from a largely descriptive field (outside of clinical trials and other clinical research studies), so that care is conducted in quantitative as well as descriptive terms. Clinical rheumatology could then have a stronger scientific basis, with accurate assessment of patient status at each visit, improved guidance for clinical monitoring, better patient outcomes, and increased respect as a quantitative clinical science.

REFERENCES

1. Pincus T, Swearingen CJ, Bergman M, et al. RAPID3 (routine assessment of patient index data 3), a rheumatoid arthritis index without formal joint counts for routine care: proposed severity categories compared to DAS and CDAI categories. J Rheumatol 2008;35:2136–47.
2. Saag KG, Teng GG, Patkar NM, et al. American College of Rheumatology 2008 recommendations for the use of nonbiologic and biologic disease-modifying antirheumatic drugs in rheumatoid arthritis. Arthritis Rheum 2008;59:762–84.
3. van der Heijde DM, van't Hof M, van Riel PL, et al. Development of a disease activity score based on judgment in clinical practice by rheumatologists. J Rheumatol 1993;20:579–81.
4. Prevoo ML, van't Hof MA, Kuper HH, et al. Modified disease activity scores that include twenty-eight-joint counts. Development and validation in a prospective longitudinal study of patients with rheumatoid arthritis. Arthritis Rheum 1995;38:44–8.
5. Aletaha D, Smolen J. The simplified disease activity index (SDAI) and the clinical disease activity index (CDAI): a review of their usefulness and validity in rheumatoid arthritis. Clin Exp Rheumatol 2005;23:S100–8.
6. Stucki G, Liang MH, Stucki S, et al. A self-administered rheumatoid arthritis disease activity index (RADAI) for epidemiologic research. Arthritis Rheum 1995;38:795–8.
7. Wolfe F, Michaud K, Pincus T. A composite disease activity scale for clinical practice, observational studies and clinical trials: the patient activity scale (PAS/PAS-II). J Rheumatol 2005;32:2410–5.
8. Yazici Y, Bergman M, Pincus T. Time to score quantitative rheumatoid arthritis measures: 28-joint count, disease activity score, health assessment questionnaire (HAQ), multidimensional HAQ (MDHAQ), and routine assessment of patient index data (RAPID) scores. J Rheumatol 2008;35:603–9.
9. Pincus T, Swearingen CJ, Bergman MJ, et al. RAPID3 on an MDHAQ is correlated significantly with activity levels of DAS28 and CDAI, but scored in 5 versus more than 90 seconds. Arthritis Care Res, in press.
10. Pincus T, Bergman MJ, Yazici Y, et al. An index of only patient-reported outcome measures, routine assessment of patient index data 3 (RAPID3), in two abatacept clinical trials: similar results to disease activity score (DAS28) and other RAPID indices that include physician-reported measures. Rheumatology (Oxford) 2008;47:345–9.
11. Pincus T, Strand V, Koch G, et al. An index of the three core data set patient questionnaire measures distinguishes efficacy of active treatment from placebo as effectively as the American College of Rheumatology 20% response criteria (ACR20) or the disease activity score (DAS) in a rheumatoid arthritis clinical trial. Arthritis Rheum 2003;48:625–30.
12. Pincus T, Chung C, Segurado OG, et al. An index of patient self-reported outcomes (PRO index) discriminates effectively between active and control treatment in 4 clinical trials of adalimumab in rheumatoid arthritis. J Rheumatol 2006; 33:2146–52.
13. Neogi T, Felson D, Niu J, et al. The association between radiographic features of knee osteoarthritis and pain: results from two cohort studies. BMJ 2009, Aug 21 [Epub ahead of print].

Complex Measures and Indices for Clinical Research Compared with Simple Patient Questionnaires to Assess Function, Pain, and Global Estimates as Rheumatology "Vital Signs" for Usual Clinical Care

Theodore Pincus, MD[a],*, Martin J. Bergman, MD[b],
Ross Maclean, MD[c], Yusuf Yazici, MD[a]

KEYWORDS

- Indices for rheumatic diseases
- Continuous quality improvement • Questionnaires • Vital signs

Pooled indices[1] have been developed to assess and monitor patient status in patients with rheumatic diseases, because a single "gold standard" such as blood pressure or cholesterol is not available for all individual patients. Indices are available to assess rheumatoid arthritis (RA),[2–20] psoriatic arthritis,[21,22] systemic lupus erythematosus (SLE),[23–30] ankylosing spondylitis,[31–36] vasculitis,[37–41] osteoarthritis,[42] fibromyalgia,[43] and other diseases (**Table 1**).[44–47] These indices generally include the 4 types of information collected in a standard medical encounter, from a patient history, physical examination, laboratory tests, and imaging studies.

A version of this article originally appeared in the 21:4 issue of *Best Practice & Research: Clinical Rheumatology*.

The work reported herein has been supported in part by the Arthritis Foundation, the Jack C. Massey Foundation, and Bristol-Myers Squibb.

[a] Division of Rheumatology, New York University School of Medicine and NYU Hospital for Joint Diseases, Room 1608, 301 East, 17th Street, New York, NY 10003, USA

[b] Division of Rheumatology, Taylor Hospital, Ridley Park, PA, USA

[c] Bristol-Myers Squibb, Princeton, NJ, USA

* Corresponding author.

E-mail address: tedpincus@gmail.com (T. Pincus).

Rheum Dis Clin N Am 35 (2009) 779–786

doi:10.1016/j.rdc.2009.10.010

0889-857X/09/$ – see front matter © 2009 Elsevier Inc. All rights reserved.

rheumatic.theclinics.com

Table 1
Measures and indices of activity or damage, or both, used to assess and monitor patients with rheumatic diseases

Disease	Indices/Measures
All rheumatic diseases	Health assessment questionnaire (HAQ)[44] HAQII[45] Multidimensional HAQ (MDHAQ)[46,47]
Rheumatoid arthritis	ACR Core Data Set[2–4] Disease activity score (DAS)[5,6] Clinical disease activity index (CDAI); simplified disease activity index (SDAI)[7] Routine assessment of patient index data 3 (RAPID3), based on 3 RA Core Data Set measures from self-report on the MDHAQ: physical function, pain, patient estimate of global status[8,9] Patient activity scale (PAS/PAS-II)[10] OMERACT criteria for minimal disease activity[11] Sharp score[12–14] van der Heijde modified sharp score[15,16] Larsen score[17–19] Ratingen score[20]
Psoriatic arthritis	ACR Core Data Set[2–4] Disease activity score (DAS)[5,6] Psoriatic arthritis response criteria (PsARC)[21] Psoriasis area and severity index (PASI)[22]
Systemic lupus erythematosus	SLE disease activity index (SLEDAI)[23] British Isles Lupus Assessment Group (BILAG) index[24] Systemic lupus activity measure (SLAM)[25] Lupus activity index (LAI)[26] European consensus lupus activity measurement (ECLAM)[27,28] SLICC/ACR damage index[30]
Ankylosing spondylitis	Bath ankylosing spondylitis disease activity index (BASDAI)[31] Modified Stoke ankylosing spondylitis spine score (mSASSS)[32] Bath ankylosing spondylitis radiology index (BASRI)[33] Bath ankylosing spondylitis functional index (BASFI)[34] Bath ankylosing spondylitis metrology index[35] Dougados functional index (DFI)[36]
Vasculitis	Birmingham vasculitis activity score (BVAS)[37] Vasculitis activity index (VAI)[38] Birmingham vasculitis damage index[40]
Wegener granulomatosis	BVAS-derived Wegener granulomatosis activity index[39] Wegener granulomatosis damage index[41]
Osteoarthritis	Western Ontario McMaster osteoarthritis index (WOMAC)[42]
Fibromyalgia	Fibromyalgia impact questionnaire (FIQ)[43]

Abbreviations: ACR, American College of Rheumatology; SLICC, Systemic Lupus International Collaborating Clinics.

Quantitative indices have led to major advances in clinical trials and other clinical research. However, excellent quantitative indices are rarely used in regular clinical care, primarily because of their complexity. Ironically, the only quantitative measures available at most regular rheumatology care visits are laboratory tests, the limitations of which led to development of composite indices in the first place. Therefore, possible benefits of important advances in quantitative measurement of rheumatic diseases to guide decisions concerning therapy, document possible effectiveness (or ineffectiveness) of these therapies, or assess quality of care are available for few, if any, patients seen in regular rheumatology care.

One perspective concerning this situation is to view development of indices largely as a research agenda. Rigorous methodologies have been applied to develop optimal validity (does the measure address what is thought to be measured?), reliability (is the measure reproducible?), and measurement precision.[48,49] However, less attention has been paid to feasibility and usefulness in usual clinical care, as is appropriate for a research activity.

Available indices are complex. Indices may include detailed quantitative physical examination measures and long self-report questionnaires (**Table 2**). The information is not amenable to being reviewed or scored easily in a busy regular clinical care setting in formulating clinical decisions. Indeed, protocols of most clinical trials and many clinical research projects direct that the investigator not review the data, but send it to a data center. Therefore, quantitative measurement seems a cumbersome burden, too complex for regular care.

Development of measures for regular clinical care involves attention not only to validity and reliability but also to feasibility, acceptability, and usefulness to patients

Table 2
Patient questionnaires for clinical research versus clinical care

(Private) Feature	Clinical Research	Clinical Care
Design considerations	Complete, long	Patient friendly, short, completed by patient within 5–10 min
Effect on patient visit	Adds time, interferes with flow	Saves time for clinician and patient
Type of questionnaire	May be "generic," "disease specific," other research goals	Applicable to patients with all rheumatic diseases
Scoring	Complex, requires computer	Simple, may "eyeball" results; scored in <20 s
Goal of data	Add to research database	Add to clinical care
Focus of analysis	Groups of patients in clinical trials or observational databases	Individual patients cared for by individual physicians
Data management	Send to data center	Review for patient care; may enter into flow-sheet to compare to previous visits
Major criteria for use	Validity, reliability; assess minimal clinically important significant difference (MCID)	Document status, medical and medicolegal rationale for aggressive therapies
Disposition of questionnaire	Enter into computer	Enter into flow sheet in medical record

and health professionals (see **Table 2**).[50–56] Patient questionnaires for usual care should be completed by most patients in 5 to 10 minutes; scanned ("eyeballed" by a clinician in 5 to 10 seconds; designed to facilitate scoring, often with scoring templates on the questionnaire; scored formally to enter into a flow sheet in 5 to 10 seconds; informative in patients with all rheumatic diseases; and may include data from a medical history and review of systems. An example of efforts to simplify measurement in rheumatology is a 28-joint count[57] in RA, scored "yes/no" for swelling and tenderness, adapted from a classic 66/68-joint count with 5 graded scores for 5 criteria: swelling, tenderness, pain on motion, deformity, and limited motion. Another example involves modification of the health assessment questionnaire (HAQ)[44] to a multidimensional HAQ (MDHAQ),[46,47] with a format designed to be reviewed, scored, and available to guide clinical decisions in busy clinical settings as noted above.

Patient questionnaires designed for standard care differ substantially from measures and indices designed for clinical trials and clinical research, and should save time for the clinician and improve the quality of patient visits.[51,58–60]

Simple scores on an MDHAQ for physical function, pain, global estimate of status, and RAPID3[8,9] may be viewed as "rheumatology vital signs" that can be collected on each patient at each visit,[61] analogous to heart rate, temperature, blood pressure, and respiration. These vital signs provide standard "scientific" data that establish a baseline, and can be compared over time. Vital signs usually confirm clinical impressions with quantitative data, but in some situations they may alert a clinician to unexpected information.

Most physicians can recognize a fever without formally measuring temperature or tachycardia without formally measuring heart rate. However, it is considerably more accurate and informative to note that "the temperature fell from 39°C to 37°C (103°F to 98.6°F)" rather than "the fever is down" or "the heart rate fell from 160 to 90" rather than "the pulse is slower." Similarly, it is considerably more accurate and informative to say that the score for pain fell from 7.5 to 2.0 rather than "the pain is improved."

Rheumatology "vital signs" are easily collected in any clinical setting. Almost all the work is done by the patient, not the physician or the staff, and the physician spends only a few valuable seconds reviewing and scoring the data.[51,52,58–60] Although the physician and patient can recognize improvement or worsening without quantitative data, quantitative data improve accuracy and are necessary to document improvement (or worsening) to another physician, payer, or any third party other than the patient or physician.

The MDHAQ also includes scales for fatigue and exercise, a review of systems, and recent medical history, which save time for the patient and physician, and improve the quality of the encounter. Comments such as "I don't have time" or "the staff would not cooperate"—among the primary reasons cited by rheumatologists for not collecting questionnaires in usual care (see "How to Collect an MDHAQ to Provide Rheumatology Vital Signs (Function, Pain, Global Status, and RAPID3 Scores) in the Infrastructure of Rheumatology Care, Including Some Misconceptions Regarding the MDHAQ," by Pincus and colleagues, in this issue)[62,63]—would be inappropriate regarding standard vital signs in an acute care setting. These comments similarly seem inappropriate reasons not to collect "rheumatology vital signs," which requires minimal effort for the physician and staff. Rheumatology vital signs should be available in the infrastructure of regular care for every visit of every patient.

REFERENCES

1. Goldsmith CH, Smythe HA, Helewa A. Interpretation and power of pooled index. J Rheumatol 1993;20:575–8.

2. van Riel PL. Provisional guidelines for measuring disease activity in clinical trials on rheumatoid arthritis [Editorial]. Br J Rheumatol 1992;31:793–4.
3. Tugwell P, Boers M. OMERACT Committee. Proceedings of the OMERACT conferences on outcome measures in rheumatoid arthritis clinical trials, Maastricht, Netherlands. J Rheumatol 1993;20:527–91.
4. Felson DT, Anderson JJ, Boers M, et al. The American college of rheumatology preliminary core set of disease activity measures for rheumatoid arthritis clinical trials. Arthritis Rheum 1993;36:729–40.
5. van der Heijde DM, van't Hof M, van Riel PL, et al. Development of a disease activity score based on judgment in clinical practice by rheumatologists. J Rheumatol 1993;20:579–81.
6. Prevoo ML, van't Hof MA, Kuper HH, et al. Modified disease activity scores that include twenty-eight-joint counts: development and validation in a prospective longitudinal study of patients with rheumatoid arthritis. Arthritis Rheum 1995;38:44–8.
7. Aletaha D, Smolen J. The simplified disease activity index (SDAI) and the clinical disease activity index (CDAI): a review of their usefulness and validity in rheumatoid arthritis. Clin Exp Rheumatol 2005;23:S100–8.
8. Pincus T, Bergman MJ, Yazici Y, et al. An index of only patient-reported outcome measures, routine assessment of patient index data 3 (RAPID3), in two abatacept clinical trials: similar results to disease activity score (DAS28) and other RAPID indices that include physician-reported measures. Rheumatology (Oxford) 2008;47:345–9.
9. Pincus T, Swearingen CJ, Bergman M, et al. RAPID3 (routine assessment of patient index data 3), a rheumatoid arthritis index without formal joint counts for routine care: proposed severity categories compared to DAS and CDAI categories. J Rheumatol 2008;35:2136–47.
10. Wolfe F, Michaud K, Pincus T. A composite disease activity scale for clinical practice, observational studies and clinical trials: the patient activity scale (PAS/PAS-II). J Rheumatol 2005;32:2410–5.
11. Wells GA, Boers M, Shea B, et al. Minimal disease activity for rheumatoid arthritis: a preliminary definition. J Rheumatol 2005;32:2016–24.
12. Sharp JT, Lidsky MD, Collins LC, et al. Methods of scoring the progression of radiologic changes in rheumatoid arthritis: correlation of radiologic, clinical and laboratory abnormalities. Arthritis Rheum 1971;14:706–20.
13. Sharp JT. Scoring radiographic abnormalities in rheumatoid arthritis. J Rheumatol 1989;16:568–9.
14. Sharp JT. Assessment of radiographic abnormalities in rheumatoid arthritis: what have we accomplished and where should we go from here? J Rheumatol 1995;22:1787–91.
15. van der Heijde D. How to read radiographs according to the Sharp/van der Heijde method. J Rheumatol 1999;26:743–5.
16. Landewe R, van der Heijde D. Radiographic progression in rheumatoid arthritis. Clin Exp Rheumatol 2005;23:S63–8.
17. Larsen A. A radiological method for grading the severity of rheumatoid arthritis [dissertation]. Helsinki (Finland): University of Helsinki; 1974.
18. Larsen A, Dale K, Eek M. Radiographic evaluation of rheumatoid arthritis and related conditions by standard reference films. Acta Radiol Diagn (Stockh) 1977;18:481–91.
19. Larsen A. How to apply Larsen score in evaluating radiographs of rheumatoid arthritis in longterm studies? J Rheumatol 1995;22:1974–5.

20. Rau R, Wassenberg S, Herborn G, et al. A new method of scoring radiographic change in rheumatoid arthritis. J Rheumatol 1998;25:2094–107.
21. Clegg DO, Reda DJ, Weisman MH, et al. Comparison of sulfasalazine and placebo in the treatment of ankylosing spondylitis. A Department of Veterans Affairs Cooperative Study. Arthritis Rheum 1996;39:2004–12.
22. Fleischer JAB, Feldman SR, Rapp SR, et al. Disease severity measures in a population of psoriasis patients: the symptoms of psoriasis correlate with self-administered psoriasis area severity index scores. J Invest Dermatol 1996;107:26–9.
23. Hawker G, Gabriel S, Bombardier C, et al. A reliability study of SLEDAI: a disease activity index for systemic lupus erythematosus. J Rheumatol 1993;20:657–60.
24. Hay EM, Bacon PA, Gordon C, et al. The BILAG index: a reliable and valid instrument for measuring clinical disease activity in systemic lupus erythematosus. Q J Med 1993;86:447–58.
25. Swaak AJ, van den Brink HG, Smeenk RJ, et al. Systemic lupus erythematosus. Disease outcome in patients with a disease duration of at least 10 years: second evaluation. Lupus 2001;10:51–8.
26. Petri M, Hellmann DB, Hochberg M. Validity and reliability of lupus activity measures in the routine clinic setting. J Rheumatol 1992;19:53–9.
27. Mosca M, Bencivelli W, Vitali C, et al. The validity of the ECLAM index for the retrospective evaluation of disease activity in systemic lupus erythematosus. Lupus 2000;9:445–50.
28. Bencivelli W, Vitali C, Isenberg DA, et al. Disease activity in systemic lupus erythematosus: report of the Consensus Study Group of the European Workshop for rheumatology research. III. Development of a computerised clinical chart and its application to the comparison of different indices of disease activity. The European Consensus Study Group for disease activity in SLE. Clin Exp Rheumatol 1992;10:549–54.
29. Gladman D, Ginzler E, Goldsmith C, et al. The development and initial validation of the Systemic Lupus International Collaborating Clinics/American College of Rheumatology Damage Index for systemic lupus erythematosus. Arthritis Rheum 1996;39:363–9.
30. Gladman DD, Urowitz MB, Goldsmith CH, et al. The reliability of the Systemic Lupus International Collaborating Clinics/American College of Rheumatology Damage Index in patients with systemic lupus erythematosus. Arthritis Rheum 1997;40:809–13.
31. Calin A, Nakache JP, Gueguen A, et al. Defining disease activity in ankylosing spondylitis: is a combination of variables (bath ankylosing spondylitis disease activity index) an appropriate instrument? Rheumatology (Oxford) 1999;38:878–82.
32. Creemers MC, Franssen MJ, van't Hof MA, et al. Assessment of outcome in ankylosing spondylitis: an extended radiographic scoring system. Ann Rheum Dis 2005;64:127–9.
33. Calin A, MacKay K, Santos H, et al. A new dimension to outcome: application of the bath ankylosing spondylitis radiology index. J Rheumatol 1999;26:988–92.
34. Calin A, Garrett S, Whitelock H, et al. A new approach to defining functional ability in ankylosing spondylitis: the development of the bath ankylosing spondylitis functional index. J Rheumatol 1994;21:2281–5.
35. Jenkinson TR, Mallorie PA, Whitelock HC, et al. Defining spinal mobility in ankylosing spondylitis (AS): the Bath AS metrology index. J Rheumatol 1994;21:1694–8.
36. Dougados M, Gueguen A, Nakache JP, et al. Evaluation of a functional index and an articular index in ankylosing spondylitis. J Rheumatol 1988;15:302–7.

37. Luqmani RA, Bacon PA, Moots RJ, et al. Birmingham Vasculitis Activity Score (BVAS) in systemic necrotizing vasculitis. Q J Med 1994;87:671–8.
38. Whiting O'Keefe QE, Stone JH, Hellmann DB. Validity of a vasculitis activity index for systemic necrotizing vasculitis. Arthritis Rheum 1999;42:2365–71.
39. Stone JH, Hoffman GS, Merkel PA, et al. A disease-specific activity index for Wegener's granulomatosis: modification of the Birmingham vasculitis activity score. Arthritis Rheum 2001;44:912–20.
40. Exley AR, Bacon PA, Luqmani RA, et al. Development and initial validation of the vasculitis damage index for the standardized clinical assessment of damage in the systemic vasculitides. Arthritis Rheum 1997;40:371–80.
41. Seo P, Min Y, Holbrook JT, et al. Damage caused by Wegener's granulomatosis and its treatment: prospective data from the Wegener's Granulomatosis Etanercept Trail (WGET). Arthritis Rheum 2005;52:2168–78.
42. Bellamy N, Buchanan WW, Goldsmith CH, et al. Validation study of WOMAC: a health status instrument for measuring clinically important patient relevant outcomes to antirheumatic drug therapy in patients with osteoarthritis of the hip or knee. J Rheumatol 1988;15:1833–40.
43. Burckhardt CS, Clark SR, Bennett RM. The fibromyalgia impact questionnaire: development and validation. J Rheumatol 1991;18:728–33.
44. Fries JF, Spitz P, Kraines RG, et al. Measurement of patient outcome in arthritis. Arthritis Rheum 1980;23:137–45.
45. Wolfe F, Michaud K, Pincus T. Development and validation of the health assessment questionnaire II: a revised version of the health assessment questionnaire. Arthritis Rheum 2004;50:3296–305.
46. Pincus T, Swearingen C, Wolfe F. Toward a multidimensional health assessment questionnaire (MDHAQ): assessment of advanced activities of daily living and psychological status in the patient friendly health assessment questionnaire format. Arthritis Rheum 1999;42:2220–30.
47. Pincus T, Sokka T, Kautiainen H. Further development of a physical function scale on a multidimensional health assessment questionnaire for standard care of patients with rheumatic diseases. J Rheumatol 2005;32:1432–9.
48. Tugwell P, Bombardier C. A methodologic framework for developing and selecting endpoints in clinical trials. J Rheumatol 1982;9:758–62.
49. Bombardier C, Tugwell P. A methodological framework to develop and select indices for clinical trials: statistical and judgmental approaches. J Rheumatol 1982;9:753–7.
50. Pincus T, Yazici Y, Bergman M. Development of a multi-dimensional health assessment questionnaire (MDHAQ) for the infrastructure of standard clinical care. Clin Exp Rheumatol 2005;23:S19–28.
51. Pincus T, Wolfe F. Patient questionnaires for clinical research and improved standard patient care: is it better to have 80% of the information in 100% of patients or 100% of the information in 5% of patients? J Rheumatol 2005;32: 575–7.
52. Pincus T, Yazici Y, Bergman M. Saving time and improving care with a multidimensional health assessment questionnaire: 10 practical considerations. J Rheumatol 2006;33:448–54.
53. Pincus T, Yazici Y, Bergman M. A practical guide to scoring a Multi-Dimensional Health Assessment Questionnaire (MDHAQ) and Routine Assessment of Patient Index Data (RAPID) scores in 10-20 seconds for use in standard clinical care, without rulers, calculators, websites or computers. Best Pract Res Clin Rheumatol 2007;21:755–87.

54. Pincus T, Yazici Y, Sokka T. Quantitative measures of rheumatic diseases for clinical research versus standard clinical care: differences, advantages and limitations. Best Pract Res Clin Rheumatol 2007;21:601–28.

55. Yazici Y, Bergman M, Pincus T. Time to score quantitative rheumatoid arthritis measures: 28-joint count, disease activity score, health assessment questionnaire (HAQ), multidimensional HAQ (MDHAQ), and routine assessment of patient index data (RAPID) scores. J Rheumatol 2008;35:603–9.

56. Pincus T, Swearingen CJ, Bergman MJ, et al. RAPID3 on an MDHAQ is correlated significantly with activity levels of DAS28 and CDAI, but scored in 5 versus more than 90 seconds. Arthritis Care Res, in press.

57. Fuchs HA, Brooks RH, Callahan LF, et al. A simplified twenty-eight joint quantitative articular index in rheumatoid arthritis. Arthritis Rheum 1989;32:531–7.

58. Pincus T, Wolfe F. An infrastructure of patient questionnaires at each rheumatology visit: improving efficiency and documenting care. J Rheumatol 2000;27:2727–30.

59. Wolfe F, Pincus T. Listening to the patient: a practical guide to self-report questionnaires in clinical care. Arthritis Rheum 1999;42:1797–808.

60. Bergmann FJ, Chassany O, Gandiol J, et al. A randomised clinical trial of the effect of informed consent on the analgesic activity of placebo and naproxen in cancer pain. Clin Trials Metaanal 1994;29:41–7.

61. Pincus T. Pain, function, and RAPID scores—vital signs in chronic diseases, analogous to pulse and temperature in acute diseases and blood pressure and cholesterol in long-term health. Bull NYU Hosp Jt Dis 2008;66:155–65.

62. Wolfe F, Pincus T, Thompson AK, et al. The assessment of rheumatoid arthritis and the acceptability of self-report questionnaires in clinical practice. Arthritis Care Res 2003;49:59–63.

63. Russak SM, Croft JD Jr, Furst DE, et al. The use of rheumatoid arthritis health-related quality of life patient questionnaire in clinical practice: lessons learned. Arthritis Rheum 2003;49:574–84.

The HAQ Compared with the MDHAQ: "Keep It Simple, Stupid" (KISS), with Feasibility and Clinical Value as Primary Criteria for Patient Questionnaires in Usual Clinical Care

Theodore Pincus, MD[a],*, Christopher J. Swearingen, PhD[b]

KEYWORDS

- Questionnaires • Health assessment questionnaire (HAQ)
- MDHAQ • RAPID3

Patient history data are more prominent in assessment and decisions concerning management of patients with rheumatic diseases than in most other types of diseases. Patient history may be captured as standardized data on self-report questionnaires. Patient questionnaires concerning functional status provide the most significant prognostic clinical measure for all important long-term outcomes of rheumatoid arthritis (RA), including functional status,[1,2] work disability,[3–5] costs,[6] joint replacement surgery,[7] and premature death.[1,8–15] Questionnaire data concerning physical function predict RA mortality at levels comparable with blood pressure, cholesterol, and smoking as risk factors for premature cardiovascular mortality.[10] However, despite

A version of this article originally appeared in the 21:4 issue of *Best Practice & Research: Clinical Rheumatology*

[a] Division of Rheumatology, Department of Medicine, New York University School of Medicine and NYU Hospital for Joint Diseases, Room 1608, 301 East 17th Street, New York, NY 10003, USA

[b] Department of Pediatrics, Biostatistics Program, University of Arkansas for Medical Sciences, Little Rock, AR, USA

* Corresponding author.
E-mail address: tedpincus@gmail.com (T. Pincus).

Rheum Dis Clin N Am 35 (2009) 787–798
doi:10.1016/j.rdc.2009.10.011
0889-857X/09/$ – see front matter © 2009 Elsevier Inc. All rights reserved.

rheumatic.theclinics.com

HEALTH ASSESSMENT QUESTIONNAIRE

ID _____ SITE_____ Date of Birth _____ Today's Date _____

This questionnaire includes information not available from blood tests, X-rays, or any source other than you. Please try to answer each question, even if you do not think it is related to you at this time. <u>There are no right or wrong answers.</u> Please answer exactly as you think or feel. Thank you.

FOR OFFICE USE ONLY

1. We are interested in learning how your illness affects your ability to function in daily life. Please check (√) the one best answer which best describes your usual abilities OVER THE PAST WEEK:

	Without ANY Difficulty(0)	With SOME Difficulty(1)	With MUCH Difficulty(2)	UNABLE To Do(3)
DRESSING & GROOMING					DRESS ☐
Are you able to:				
- Dress yourself, including tying shoelaces and doing buttons?	____	____	____	____
- Shampoo your hair?	____	____	____	____	ARISE ☐
ARISING				
Are you able to:				
- Stand up from a straight chair?	____	____	____	____
- Get in and out of bed?	____	____	____	____
EATING					EAT ☐
Are you able to:				
- Cut your meat?	____	____	____	____
- Lift a full cup or glass to your mouth?	____	____	____	____
- Open a new milk carton?	____	____	____	____
WALKING					WALK ☐
Are you able to:				
- Walk outdoors on flat ground?	____	____	____	____
- Climb up five steps?	____	____	____	____

2. Please check any **AIDS OR DEVICES** that you usually use for any of these activities:

_____ Cane   _____ Devices used for dressing (button hook, zipper pull, long-handled shoe horn, etc.)

_____ Walker   _____ Built up or special utensils

_____ Crutches   _____ Special or built up chair

_____ Wheelchair   _____ Other (Specify: _____)

ASST
Drsg____
Rise____
Eat____
Walk____

3. Please check any categories for which you usually need **HELP FROM ANOTHER PERSON:**

_____ Dressing and Grooming   _____ Eating

_____ Arising   _____ Walking

4. How much pain have you had **OVER THE PAST WEEK?** Place a mark on the line below to indicate how severe your pain has been:

PAIN ☐

NO PAIN |————————————————————————————| PAIN AS BAD AS IT COULD BE

Fig. 1. Health assessment questionnaire (HAQ). (*From* Fries JF, Spitz P, Kraines RG, et al. Measurement of patient outcome in arthritis. Arthritis Rheum 1980;23:137–45; with permission.)

their value in assessment, monitoring, and prognosis, patient questionnaires have been incorporated into only a minority of standard rheumatology care settings.

The most widely used patient questionnaire in rheumatology is the health assessment questionnaire (HAQ) (**Fig. 1**).[16] The HAQ and the arthritis impact measurement scale (AIMS)[16] were first reported in 1980. The senior author, who has a strong interest in clinical measurement,[17,18] began using these questionnaires for patient assessment

5. **Please check the response which best describes your usual abilities OVER THE PAST WEEK:**

	Without ANY Difficulty(0)	With SOME Difficulty(1)	With MUCH Difficulty(2)	UNABLE To Do(3)	FOR OFFICE USE ONLY
HYGIENE					
Are you able to:					
- Wash and dry your body?	___	___	___	___	HYG ☐
- Take a tub bath?	___	___	___	___	
- Get on and off the toilet?	___	___	___	___	
REACH					
Are you able to:					
- Reach and get down a 5 pound object (such as a bag of sugar) from just above your head?	___	___	___	___	REACH ☐
- Bend down to pick up clothing from the floor?	___	___	___	___	
GRIP					
Are you able to:					
- Open car doors?	___	___	___	___	GRIP ☐
- Open jars which have previously been opened?	___	___	___	___	
- Turn faucets on and off?	___	___	___	___	
ACTIVITIES					
Are you able to:					
- Run errands and shop?	___	___	___	___	ACT ☐
- Get in and out of a car?	___	___	___	___	
- Do chores such as vacuuming or yard work?	___	___	___	___	

6. **Please check any AIDS OR DEVICES that you usually use for any of these activities:**

____ Raised toilet seat   ____ Bathtub bar
____ Bathtub seat   ____ Long-handled appliances for reach
____ Jar opener (for jars previously opened)   ____ Long-handled appliances in bathroom
____ Other (Specify: _____)

ASST
Hyg____
Rch____
Grip____
Act____

7. **Please check any categories for which you usually need HELP FROM ANOTHER PERSON:**

____ Hygiene   ____ Gripping and opening things
____ Reach   ____ Errands and chores

8. **Considering all the ways in which illness and health conditions may affect you at this time, please make a mark below to show how you are doing:**

GLOB ☐

VERY WELL |———————————————————————————| VERY POORLY

Fig. 1. (*continued*)

in routine care at that time. Over a few months, it became apparent that the HAQ was far more "patient friendly" than the AIMS questionnaire for standard care although the AIMS had superior psychometric properties, and the HAQ became the only questionnaire used.

The HAQ (see **Fig. 1**) lists 20 activities grouped into 8 categories of 2 or 3 activities each: dressing and grooming, arising, eating, walking, hygiene, reach, grip, and activities. Each item is scored on a scale of 0 to 3 (0 = without any difficulty, 1 = with some difficulty, 2 = with much difficulty, 3 = unable to do). The HAQ includes queries about "help from another person" and "use of aids and devices" in any of these categories. The score is increased by 1, or scored as 2 (different versions exist), if "aids or devices" or "help from another person" is used. The HAQ also includes two 10-cm visual analog scales (VAS) scored 0 to 10 to assess pain and patient global estimate of status.

Multi-Dimensional Health Assessment Questionnaire (R808-NP2)

This questionnaire includes information not available from blood tests, X-rays, or any source other than you. Please try to answer each question, even if you do not think it is related to you at this time. Try to complete as much as you can yourself, but if you need help, please ask. There are no right or wrong answers. Please answer exactly as you think or feel. Thank you.

1. Please check (√) the ONE best answer for your abilities at this time:

OVER THE LAST WEEK, were you able to:	Without ANY Difficulty	With SOME Difficulty	With MUCH Difficulty	UNABLE To Do
a. Dress yourself, including tying shoelaces and doing buttons?	0	1	2	3
b. Get in and out of bed?	0	1	2	3
c. Lift a full cup or glass to your mouth?	0	1	2	3
d. Walk outdoors on flat ground?	0	1	2	3
e. Wash and dry your entire body?	0	1	2	3
f. Bend down to pick up clothing from the floor?	0	1	2	3
g. Turn regular faucets on and off?	0	1	2	3
h. Get in and out of a car, bus, train, or airplane?	0	1	2	3
i. Walk two miles or three kilometers, if you wish?	0	1	2	3
j. Participate in recreational activities and sports as you would like, if you wish?	0	1	2	3
k. Get a good night's sleep?	0	1.1	2.2	3.3
l. Deal with feelings of anxiety or being nervous?	0	1.1	2.2	3.3
m. Deal with feelings of depression or feeling blue?	0	1.1	2.2	3.3

FOR OFFICE USE ONLY

1.a-j FN (0-10):

1=0.3 16=5.3
2=0.7 17=5.7
3=1.0 18=6.0
4=1.3 19=6.3
5=1.7 20=6.7
6=2.0 21=7.0
7=2.3 22=7.3
8=2.7 23=7.7
9=3.0 24=8.0
10=3.3 25=8.3
11=3.7 26=8.7
12=4.0 27=9.0
13=4.3 28=9.3
14=4.7 29=9.7
15=5.0 30=10

2.PN (0-10):

2. How much pain have you had because of your condition OVER THE PAST WEEK? Please indicate below how severe your pain has been:

NO PAIN 0 0.5 1.0 1.5 2.0 2.5 3.0 3.5 4.0 4.5 5.0 5.5 6.0 6.5 7.0 7.5 8.0 8.5 9.0 9.5 10 PAIN AS BAD AS IT COULD BE

4.PTGL (0-10):

RAPID 3 (0-30):

3. Please place a check (√) in the appropriate spot to indicate the amount of pain you are having today in each of the joint areas listed below:

	None	Mild	Moderate	Severe		None	Mild	Moderate	Severe
a. LEFT FINGERS	□0	□1	□2	□3	i. RIGHT FINGERS	□0	□1	□2	□3
b. LEFT WRIST	□0	□1	□2	□3	j. RIGHT WRIST	□0	□1	□2	□3
c. LEFT ELBOW	□0	□1	□2	□3	k. RIGHT ELBOW	□0	□1	□2	□3
d. LEFT SHOULDER	□0	□1	□2	□3	l. RIGHT SHOULDER	□0	□1	□2	□3
e. LEFT HIP	□0	□1	□2	□3	m. RIGHT HIP	□0	□1	□2	□3
f. LEFT KNEE	□0	□1	□2	□3	n. RIGHT KNEE	□0	□1	□2	□3
g. LEFT ANKLE	□0	□1	□2	□3	o. RIGHT ANKLE	□0	□1	□2	□3
h. LEFT TOES	□0	□1	□2	□3	p. RIGHT TOES	□0	□1	□2	□3
q. NECK	□0	□1	□2	□3	r. BACK	□0	□1	□2	□3

Cat:

HS = >12

MS = 6.1-12

LS = 3.1-6

R = ≤3

4. Considering all the ways in which illness and health conditions may affect you at this time, please indicate below how you are doing:

VERY WELL 0 0.5 1.0 1.5 2.0 2.5 3.0 3.5 4.0 4.5 5.0 5.5 6.0 6.5 7.0 7.5 8.0 8.5 9.0 9.5 10 VERY POORLY

Fig. 2. Multidimensional health assessment questionnaire (MDHAQ). The front page (A) includes 10 activities for function and 2 visual analog scales (VAS) for pain and patient global estimate of status, and a self-report joint count from a rheumatoid arthritis disease activity index (RADAI). Scoring templates for these measures are available on the right-hand edge of the page. An index of the 3 patient-reported measures, routine assessment of patient index data (RAPID3), can be calculated from an MDHAQ in fewer than 10 seconds. The reverse side (B) includes a review of systems, fatigue VAS, queries regarding morning stiffness, change in status, exercise, recent medical history, and demographic data (not included in scoring, but providing useful data in clinical care). (Copyright © 2009 Health Report Services, Inc. Email: tedpincus@gmail.com.)

Activities on the HAQ are listed on 2 pages (2 sides of one sheet of paper), rendering a quick "eyeball" scan in the clinic difficult. Some activities on the HAQ, for example, "shampoo your hair" and "run errands," are not performed by some individuals. Scoring the HAQ physical function scale is somewhat complex, ultimately shown to require 42 seconds.[19]

5. Please check (√) if you have experienced any of the following <u>over the last month:</u>

			FOR OFFICE
__Fever	__Lump in your throat	__Paralysis of arms or legs	USE ONLY
__Weight gain (>10 lbs)	__Cough	__Numbness or tingling of arms or legs	
__Weight loss (>10 lbs)	__Shortness of breath	__Fainting spells	5. ROS:
__Feeling sickly	__Wheezing	__Swelling of hands	
__Headaches	__Pain in the chest	__Swelling of ankles	□
__Unusual fatigue	__Heart pounding (palpitations)	__Swelling in other joints	
__Swollen glands	__Trouble swallowing	__Joint pain	

__Fever — __Lump in your throat — __Paralysis of arms or legs
__Weight gain (>10 lbs) — __Cough — __Numbness or tingling of arms or legs
__Weight loss (>10 lbs) — __Shortness of breath — __Fainting spells
__Feeling sickly — __Wheezing — __Swelling of hands
__Headaches — __Pain in the chest — __Swelling of ankles
__Unusual fatigue — __Heart pounding (palpitations) — __Swelling in other joints
__Swollen glands — __Trouble swallowing — __Joint pain
__Loss of appetite — __Heartburn or stomach gas — __Back pain
__Skin rash or hives — __Stomach pain or cramps — __Neck pain
__Unusual bruising or bleeding — __Nausea — __Use of drugs not sold in stores
__Other skin problems — __Vomiting — __Smoking cigarettes
__Loss of hair — __Constipation — __More than 2 alcoholic drinks per day
__Dry eyes — __Diarrhea — __Depression - feeling blue
__Other eye problems — __Dark or bloody stools — __Anxiety - feeling nervous
__Problems with hearing — __Problems with urination — __Problems with thinking
__Ringing in the ears — __Gynecological (female) problems — __Problems with memory
__Stuffy nose — __Dizziness — __Problems with sleeping
__Sores in the mouth — __Losing your balance — __Sexual problems
__Dry mouth — __Muscle pain, aches, or cramps — __Burning in sex organs
__Problems with smell or taste — __Muscle weakness — __Problems with social activities

Please check (√) here if you have had none of the above over the last month: _____.

6. When you awakened in the morning OVER THE LAST WEEK, did you feel stiff? □ No □ Yes
If "No," please go to Item 7. If "Yes," please indicate the number of minutes_____, or hours _____ until you are as limber as you will be for the day.

7. How do you feel TODAY compared to ONE WEEK AGO? Please check (✓) only one.
Much Better □ (1), Better □ (2), the Same □ (3), Worse □ (4), Much Worse □ (5) than one week ago

8. How often do you exercise aerobically (sweating, increased heart rate, shortness of breath) for at least one-half hour (30 minutes)? Please check (✓) only one.
□ 3 or more times a week (3)   □ 1-2 times per month (1)
□ 1-2 times per week   (2)   □ Do not exercise regularly (0)   □ Cannot exercise due to disability/ handicap (9)

9. How much of a problem has UNUSUAL fatigue or tiredness been for you OVER THE PAST WEEK?
FATIGUE IS ○ FATIGUE IS A
NO PROBLEM 0 0.5 1.0 1.5 2.0 2.5 3.0 3.5 4.0 4.5 5.0 5.5 6.0 6.5 7.0 7.5 8.0 8.5 9.0 9.5 10   MAJOR PROBLEM

10. Over the last 6 months have you had: [Please check (√)]
□No □Yes An operation or new illness   □No □Yes Change(s) of arthritis or other medication
□No □Yes Medical emergency or stay overnight in hospital   □No □Yes Change(s) of address
□No □Yes A fall, broken bone, or other accident or trauma   □No □Yes Change(s) of marital status
□No □Yes An important new symptom or medical problem   □No □Yes Change job or work duties, quit work, retired
□No □Yes Side effect(s) of any medication or drug   □No □Yes Change of medical insurance, Medicare, etc.
□No □Yes Smoke cigarettes regularly   □No □Yes Change of primary care or other doctor
Please explain any "Yes" answer below, or indicate any other health matter that affects you:
_____
_____

SEX: □ Female, □ Male ETHNIC GROUP: □ Asian, □ Black, □ Hispanic, □ White, □ Other_____

Your Occupation _____ Please circle the number of years of school you have completed:
Work Status: □ Full-time, □ Part-time, □ Disabled   1 2 3 4 5 6 7 8 9 10
□ Homemaker, □ Self-Employed, □Retired,   11 12 13 14 15 16 17 18 19 20
□ Seeking work, □ Other_____ Please write your weight: _____ lbs. height: _____ inches

Your Name_____ Date of Birth _____ Today's Date _____

Page 2 of 2 Thank you for completing this questionnaire to help keep track of your medical care.   R808NP2

FOR OFFICE USE ONLY: I have reviewed the questionnaire responses.
Date: _____ Signature_____

Fig. 2. (continued)

These considerations led to development of a modified HAQ (MHAQ) in the early 1980s,[20] which included only one activity from each of the 8 HAQ categories, chosen among activities that all individuals would perform each day. "Aids and devices" and "help from another person" were deleted. All 8 activities, as well as the VAS for pain and patient global estimate, were found on one side of a sheet of paper, facilitating "eyeball" review in the clinic by the physician.

In 1982, analyses of a cohort of patients with RA over 9 years indicated that patient questionnaire data concerning physical function were the most significant predictor of premature mortality.[1,10,21] This observation has been replicated in 17 of 18 RA cohorts analyzed for long-term mortality,[15] in which patient questionnaire data have far greater

Multi-Dimensional Health Assessment Questionnaire (R811-NP4)

This questionnaire includes information not available from blood tests, X-rays, or any source other than you. Please try to answer each question, even if you do not think it is related to you at this time. Try to complete as much as you can yourself, but if you need help, please ask. There are no right or wrong answers.   Please answer exactly as you think or feel. Thank you.

1. Please check (√) the ONE best answer for your abilities at this time:

OVER THE LAST WEEK, were you able to:	Without ANY Difficulty	With SOME Difficulty	With MUCH Difficulty	UNABLE To Do
a. Dress yourself, including tying shoelaces and doing buttons?	0	1	2	3
b. Get in and out of bed?	0	1	2	3
c. Lift a full cup or glass to your mouth?	0	1	2	3
d. Walk outdoors on flat ground?	0	1	2	3
e. Wash and dry your entire body?	0	1	2	3
f. Bend down to pick up clothing from the floor?	0	1	2	3
g. Turn regular faucets on and off?	0	1	2	3
h. Get in and out of a car, bus, train, or airplane?	0	1	2	3
i. Walk two miles or three kilometers, if you wish?	0	1	2	3
j. Participate in recreational activities and sports as you would like, if you wish?	0	1	2	3
k. Get a good night's sleep?	0	1.1	2.2	3.3
l. Deal with feelings of anxiety or being nervous?	0	1.1	2.2	3.3
m. Deal with feelings of depression or feeling blue?	0	1.1	2.2	3.3

FOR OFFICE USE ONLY

1.a-j FN (0-10):

1=0.3	16=5.3
2=0.7	17=5.7
3=1.0	18=6.0
4=1.3	19=6.3
5=1.7	20=6.7
6=2.0	21=7.0
7=2.3	22=7.3
8=2.7	23=7.7
9=3.0	24=8.0
10=3.3	25=8.3
11=3.7	26=8.7
12=4.0	27=9.0
13=4.3	28=9.3
14=4.7	29=9.7
15=5.0	30=10

2. How much pain have you had because of your condition OVER THE PAST WEEK? Please indicate below how severe your pain has been:

NO ○ PAIN AS BAD AS
PAIN 0 0.5 1.0 1.5 2.0 2.5 3.0 3.5 4.0 4.5 5.0 5.5 6.0 6.5 7.0 7.5 8.0 8.5 9.0 9.5 10 IT COULD BE

2.PN (0-10):

4.PTGL (0-10):

RAPID 3 (0-30):

3. Please place a check (√) in the appropriate spot to indicate the amount of pain you are having today in each of the joint areas listed below:

	None	Mild	Moderate	Severe		None	Mild	Moderate	Severe
a. LEFT FINGERS	☐0	☐1	☐2	☐3	i. RIGHT FINGERS	☐0	☐1	☐2	☐3
b. LEFT WRIST	☐0	☐1	☐2	☐3	j. RIGHT WRIST	☐0	☐1	☐2	☐3
c. LEFT ELBOW	☐0	☐1	☐2	☐3	k. RIGHT ELBOW	☐0	☐1	☐2	☐3
d. LEFT SHOULDER	☐0	☐1	☐2	☐3	l. RIGHT SHOULDER	☐0	☐1	☐2	☐3
e. LEFT HIP	☐0	☐1	☐2	☐3	m. RIGHT HIP	☐0	☐1	☐2	☐3
f. LEFT KNEE	☐0	☐1	☐2	☐3	n. RIGHT KNEE	☐0	☐1	☐2	☐3
g. LEFT ANKLE	☐0	☐1	☐2	☐3	o. RIGHT ANKLE	☐0	☐1	☐2	☐3
h. LEFT TOES	☐0	☐1	☐2	☐3	p. RIGHT TOES	☐0	☐1	☐2	☐3
q. NECK	☐0	☐1	☐2	☐3	r. BACK	☐0	☐1	☐2	☐3

Cat:
HS = >12
MS = 6.1-12
LS = 3.1-6
R = <3

4. Considering all the ways in which illness and health conditions may affect you at this time, please indicate below how you are doing:

VERY ○ VERY
WELL 0 0.5 1.0 1.5 2.0 2.5 3.0 3.5 4.0 4.5 5.0 5.5 6.0 6.5 7.0 7.5 8.0 8.5 9.0 9.5 10 POORLY

Fig. 3. (A–D) A 4-page (2 sheets of paper) version of the MDHAQ designed for the new patient/ initial visit. (Copyright © 2009 Health Report Services, Inc. Email: tedpincus@gmail.com.)

significance than laboratory or radiographic data in predicting mortality.[15] The finding of high prognostic significance of questionnaire data for premature mortality in RA is consistent with the prominence of patient-reported information in standard rheumatology care, compared with care of patients with other diseases. These observations transformed the patient self-report questionnaire from an "elective" measure to status as a "required" measure, to be completed by each patient at each visit in the usual care of the senior author.

The choice of simple activities performed daily by all people, in selecting 8 items from the HAQ for inclusion in the MHAQ, led to systematically lower scores compared with the HAQ, by about 0.3 units on a scale of 0 to 3, or 10%.[22] This finding, along with the improving status of patients with rheumatic diseases,[23] led in the mid-1990s to the

5. Please check (√) if you have experienced any of the following <u>over the last month</u>:

__Fever	__Lump in your throat	__Paralysis of arms or legs	**FOR OFFICE USE ONLY**
__Weight gain (>10 lbs)	__Cough	__Numbness or tingling of arms or legs	
__Weight loss (>10 lbs)	__Shortness of breath	__Fainting spells	**5. ROS:**
__Feeling sickly	__Wheezing	__Swelling of hands	
__Headaches	__Pain in the chest	__Swelling of ankles	☐
__Unusual fatigue	__Heart pounding (palpitations)	__Swelling in other joints	
__Swollen glands	__Trouble swallowing	__Joint pain	
__Loss of appetite	__Heartburn or stomach gas	__Back pain	
__Skin rash or hives	__Stomach pain or cramps	__Neck pain	
__Unusual bruising or bleeding	__Nausea	__Use of drugs not sold in stores	
__Other skin problems	__Vomiting	__Smoking cigarettes	
__Loss of hair	__Constipation	__More than 2 alcoholic drinks per day	
__Dry eyes	__Diarrhea	__Depression - feeling blue	
__Other eye problems	__Dark or bloody stools	__Anxiety - feeling nervous	
__Problems with hearing	__Problems with urination	__Problems with thinking	
__Ringing in the ears	__Gynecological (female) problems	__Problems with memory	
__Stuffy nose	__Dizziness	__Problems with sleeping	
__Sores in the mouth	__Losing your balance	__Sexual problems	
__Dry mouth	__Muscle pain, aches, or cramps	__Burning in sex organs	
__Problems with smell or taste	__Muscle weakness	__Problems with social activities	

Please check (√) here if you have had none of the above over the last month: _____.

6. When you awakened in the morning OVER THE LAST WEEK, did you feel stiff? ☐ No   ☐ Yes
If "No," please go to Item 7. If "Yes," please indicate the number of minutes_____, or hours _____ until you are as limber as you will be for the day.

7. How do you feel TODAY compared to ONE WEEK AGO? Please check (✓) only one.
Much Better ☐ (1),   Better ☐ (2),   the Same ☐ (3),   Worse ☐ (4),   Much Worse ☐ (5) than one week ago

8. How often do you exercise aerobically (sweating, increased heart rate, shortness of breath) **for at least one-half hour** (30 minutes)? **Please check (✓) only one.**

☐ 3 or more times a week (3)   ☐ 1-2 times per month (1)
☐ 1-2 times per week   (2)   ☐ Do not exercise regularly (0)   ☐ Cannot exercise due to disability/ handicap (9)

9. How much of a problem has UNUSUAL fatigue or tiredness been for you OVER THE PAST WEEK?

FATIGUE IS   ○   FATIGUE IS A
NO PROBLEM   0 0.5 1.0 1.5 2.0 2.5 3.0 3.5 4.0 4.5 5.0 5.5 6.0 6.5 7.0 7.5 8.0 8.5 9.0 9.5 10   MAJOR PROBLEM

10. Over the last 6 months have you had: [Please check (√)]

☐No ☐Yes An operation or new illness	☐No ☐Yes	Change(s) of arthritis or other medication
☐No ☐Yes Medical emergency or stay overnight in hospital	☐No ☐Yes	Change(s) of address
☐No ☐Yes A fall, broken bone, or other accident or trauma	☐No ☐Yes	Change(s) of marital status
☐No ☐Yes An important new symptom or medical problem	☐No ☐Yes	Change job or work duties, quit work, retired
☐No ☐Yes Side effect(s) of any medication or drug	☐No ☐Yes	Change of medical insurance, Medicare, etc.
☐No ☐Yes Smoke cigarettes regularly	☐No ☐Yes	Change of primary care or other doctor

Please explain any "Yes" answer below, or indicate any other health matter that affects you:

_____

_____

11. Please list below any medications which you cannot take because you are allergic to them:

_____   _____   _____   _____

12. Please list below anything else (grass, molds, pollens, etc.) you might be allergic to:

_____   _____   _____   _____

Fig. 3. (*continued*)

addition of complex activities into what is now known as a multidimensional HAQ (MDHAQ) (**Fig. 2**).[22] The MDHAQ includes 10 activities, 8 from the MHAQ (and HAQ), and 2 complex activities: "Are you able to walk 2 miles or 3 kilometers?" and "Are you able to participate in recreational activities and sports as you would like?" Scores on the MDHAQ are similar to the HAQ.[22,24]

Two versions of the MDHAQ are available: R808, a 2-page questionnaire (single sheet of paper) that may be used for "new" or "return" patients (see **Fig. 2**), and R811, a 4-page version for new patients (**Fig. 3**). **Table 1** lists the features of the MDHAQ that have been introduced over 29 years to facilitate clinical care, save time for the physician, and improve the quality, documentation, and outcomes of patient care.

13. Please check (✓) either "No" or "Yes" to indicate whether or not you have any of the conditions below:
Have you ever had: **If you answer "Yes", please list AGE or YEAR when it began.**

			AGE or YEAR				**AGE or YEAR**
High Blood Pressure or				Gynecological (Female)/			
Hypertension	__No	__Yes	___ or ___	Prostate (Male) problem	__No	__Yes	___ or ___
Heart attack	__No	__Yes	___ or ___	Severe allergies	__No	__Yes	___ or ___
Other heart disease	__No	__Yes	___ or ___	Rheumatoid arthritis	__No	__Yes	___ or ___
Cancer	__No	__Yes	___ or ___	Osteoarthritis	__No	__Yes	___ or ___
Stroke	__No	__Yes	___ or ___	Lupus	__No	__Yes	___ or ___
Bronchitis or Emphysema	__No	__Yes	___ or ___	Back or spine problems	__No	__Yes	___ or ___
Asthma	__No	__Yes	___ or ___	Fibromyalgia (Fibrositis)	__No	__Yes	___ or ___
Other Lung problem	__No	__Yes	___ or ___	Osteoporosis	__No	__Yes	___ or ___
Anemia (Low Blood)	__No	__Yes	___ or ___	Broken bones after age 50	__No	__Yes	___ or ___
Other hematologic problem	__No	__Yes	___ or ___	Dry mouth	__No	__Yes	___ or ___
Stomach ulcer	__No	__Yes	___ or ___	Dry eyes	__No	__Yes	___ or ___
Other gastrointestinal				Cataracts	__No	__Yes	___ or ___
(GI) problem	__No	__Yes	___ or ___	Parkinson's disease	__No	__Yes	___ or ___
Thyroid problem	__No	__Yes	___ or ___	Depression	__No	__Yes	___ or ___
Diabetes	__No	__Yes	___ or ___	Mental illness	__No	__Yes	___ or ___
Kidney problem	__No	__Yes	___ or ___	Alcoholism	__No	__Yes	___ or ___

Other _____ ___ or ___   Other _____ ___ or ___
     (Please name)   (Please name)

14. Please list below all operations you have ever had. Please check (✓) here if none: _____.

	Operation	Year	Surgeon	Hospital, City, State
1.				
2.				
3.				
4.				

(You may continue below or on a separate page)

15. Please list below all major illnesses or hospital admissions (other than for operations).
Please check (✓) here if none: _____.

	Illness or Reason for hospitalization	Year	Hospital, City, State
1.			
2.			
3.			
4.			

(You may continue below or on a separate page)

16. The questions below concern your family medical history:

	If Living		If Deceased	
	Birth Year or Age	Any Major Medical Conditions	Year or Age at death	Cause(s) of death
Father				
Mother				
Brother(s)				
Sister(s)				
Son(s)				
Daughter(s)				

17. Any blood relative (parent, child, brother, sister, aunt, uncle) with: If "Yes", give relationship.

	No	Yes	Relation(s)		No	Yes	Relation(s)
Rheumatoid Arthritis	__	__	_____	Lupus or SLE	__	__	_____

18. Any illnesses which run in the family? _____

Fig. 3. (*continued*)

Page 1 of the MDHAQ includes 4 scales to assess physical function (FN), pain (PN), rheumatoid arthritis disease activity index (RADAI),[25] self-report joint count (PTJT), and patient global status (PTGL). The 10 activities of the physical function scale are each scored 0 to 3, for a total of 0 to 30; a scoring template ("For Office Use Only") facilitates calculation of physical function, with division of the 0 to 30 scale by 3 to provide a 0 to 10 score. The VAS for pain and patient global estimate consist of 21 numbered circles[26] rather than a 10-cm line on the HAQ; this change allows the physician to score these scales instantly, without using a ruler to measure the point from the origin to score these scales (as required on the HAQ and MHAQ). Boxes are available at the right side to enter scores for physical function, pain, and patient global estimate, each scored 0 to 10. A composite RAPID3 score ranges from 0 to 30, and can be scored in 5 to 10 seconds.[19,27]

19. **Please write below all pills that you took over the last TWO WEEKS, with or without a prescription.** Include aspirin, birth control pills, pain pills, alternative therapy, health supplements, pills sold in health food stores:

NAME OF DRUG, MEDICINE OR ALTERNATIVE THERAPY	DOSE (if known)	How Many per day or week?	NAME OF DRUG, MEDICINE OR ALTERNATIVE THERAPY	DOSE (if known)	How Many Per day or week?
1.			7.		
2.			8.		
3.			9.		
4.			10.		
5.			11.		
6.			12.		

20. **What is your current occupation?** (If you are not working now, what was your past occupation?)

_____

21. **At this time, are you?**[Please check(✓)all that apply.]
__Working full time   __Retired
__Working part time   __Student
__Homemaker-full time   __Disabled
__Seeking work   __Other (describe)_____

22. **How many other people live at home with you?** ___
[Please check (✓) who lives with you.]
__Spouse/partner   __Parents   __Sons or daughters
__I live alone   __Others (describe)_____

23. **How many years of school have you completed?**
Please circle the number of years of school:
1 2 3 4 5 6 7 8 9 10
11 12 13 14 15 16 17 18 19 20

24. **Please write your weight:** ____lbs. height: ___in.

Your Name_____   Today's Date_____   Time of Day____ AM/PM
        First   Middle   Last

Street Address_____ City_____ State____ Zip_____

Telephone (__) _____ Social Security #_____ Date of Birth _____
    Area Code   Number   For Identification Purposes Only

SEX: ☐ Female   ETHNIC ☐ Asian ☐ Hispanic ☐ Other   MARITAL STATUS: ☐ Single   ☐ Married   ☐ Divorced
    ☐ Male   GROUP: ☐ Black ☐ White   ☐ Widowed   ☐ Separated

Please check if this questionnaire is completed ☐ **entirely by patient** OR ☐ **with help from (name)**_____

WE ASK YOU FOR CONSENT TO REVIEW YOUR RECORDS FOR MEDICAL RESEARCH AND TO CONTACT YOU IN THE FUTURE. YOUR CARE WILL NOT BE AFFECTED IF YOU ANSWER "NO."
I agree to allow information from my medical record to be reviewed for medical research, and for you to send me similar questionnaires in the future, which I am not required to answer. I understand that this information will remain confidential with my doctor and his or her research associates only. Please check (✓) in **one** box. Thank you!

☐ YES   ☐ NO   Signature_____   Date _____

I understand and agree that my doctor may share this information with colleagues at other medical research centers, in order to learn more about best treatments for my condition. Please check (✓) in **one** box. Thank you!

☐ YES   ☐ NO   Signature_____   Date _____

Please list the name, address, and telephone number of your primary care physician:
Name_____   Address_____
City, State ZIP _____   Telephone _____

Please list the name of your rheumatologist and insurance center:
Rheumatologist_____   Insurance_____

Please list the name, address, and telephone number of someone who lives at a different address from you, and who will be likely to know your whereabouts if we are unable to reach you:
Name_____   Address_____
City, State ZIP _____   Telephone_____ Relationship _____

Page 4 of 4   Thank you for completing this questionnaire to help keep track of your medical care.   R811NP4

| FOR OFFICE USE ONLY: I have reviewed the questionnaire responses. |
| Date: _____   Signature_____ |

Fig. 3. (continued)

The inclusion of the RADAI self-report joint count[25] is helpful to the clinicians, particularly for a medical record note—typed or dictated. The RADAI also separates the VAS for pain from the VAS for global estimate, on the page, to reduce the likelihood that a patient would enter identical scores for both VAS, although these scores are highly correlated, as pain is a primary determinant of global status in most patients. Scoring of the RADAI on a 0 to 10 scale was described in earlier reports.[28] However, scores that included a RADAI self-report joint count or physician/assessor joint count were so similar to RAPID3 scores without a joint count[28,29] that scoring of the RADAI is no longer advocated (see "RAPID3, an Index to Assess and Monitor Patients with

Table 1
Comparison of the health assessment questionnaire (HAQ)[16] and multidimensional HAQ (MDHAQ)[22]

	HAQ	MDHAQ
First report	1980	1999
Patient completion	5–10 min	5–10 min
# ADL	20	10
Pain VAS	10-cm line	21 circles
Patient global VAS	10-cm line	21 circles
Psych, sleep	No	Sleep, anxiety, depression
RADAI self-report joint count[25]	No	Yes
Fatigue	No	VAS
Review of systems	No	60 symptoms
Medical history	No	Surgery, side effects
Demographic data	No	Yes
Social history	No	Yes
Scoring templates	No	Yes
Index	No	RAPID3
MD scan ("eyeball")	30 s	5 s
Time to score	42 s	5 s

Rheumatoid Arthritis, Without Formal Joint Counts: Similar Results to DAS28 and CDAI in Clinical Trials and Clinical Care," by Pincus and colleagues, in this issue).

Page 2 of the MDHAQ includes a review of systems (ROS) in the form of a 60-symptom checklist, with a box to enter the actual number of symptoms checked. As discussed elsewhere (see "Clues on the MDHAQ to Identify Patients with Fibromyalgia and Similar Chronic Pain Conditions," by Pincus and colleagues, in this issue), a report of more than 20 symptoms is characteristic of patients with fibromyalgia or chronic pain syndrome, but not of patients with RA or other inflammatory diseases.[30] This observation may be regarded as providing quantitative documentation of a "positive review of systems" with a quantitative "scientific" score. The score can be particularly helpful in patients who have an inflammatory disease such as RA or systemic lupus erythematosus and also have fibromyalgia, about 20%"to 30% of patients with RA.[31] Page 2 also includes queries concerning morning stiffness, change in status, exercise, VAS for fatigue (0–10 scale), a series of 12 "yes/no" questions concerning recent medical history, demographic data, and social history. The recent medical history was found to save 2 to 3 minutes at most encounters.

The 4-page version of the MDHAQ for new patients (see **Fig. 3**) also includes a recent medical history, surgeries, family history, allergies, and medications. The 4-page MDHAQ facilitates an approach to quality control of a medical history in a database or electronic medical record, with participation of the patient as a partner (see "Quality Control of a Medical History: Improving Accuracy with Patient Participation, Supported by a Four-Page Version of the Multidimensional Health Assessment Questionnaire (MDHAQ)," by Pincus and colleagues, in this issue). Although the HAQ can be used in usual care, features of the MDHAQ include scoring RAPID3 in 5 to 10 seconds rather than 42 seconds. The MDHAQ may include more features for usual clinical care.

REFERENCES

1. Pincus T, Callahan LF, Sale WG, et al. Severe functional declines, work disability, and increased mortality in seventy-five rheumatoid arthritis patients studied over nine years. Arthritis Rheum 1984;27:864–72.
2. Wolfe F, Cathey MA. The assessment and prediction of functional disability in rheumatoid arthritis. J Rheumatol 1991;18:1298–306.
3. Callahan LF, Bloch DA, Pincus T. Identification of work disability in rheumatoid arthritis: physical, radiographic and laboratory variables do not add explanatory power to demographic and functional variables. J Clin Epidemiol 1992;45:127–38.
4. Wolfe F, Hawley DJ. The longterm outcomes of rheumatoid arthritis: work disability: a prospective 18 year study of 823 patients. J Rheumatol 1998;25:2108–17.
5. Sokka T, Kautiainen H, Möttönen T, et al. Work disability in rheumatoid arthritis 10 years after the diagnosis. J Rheumatol 1999;26:1681–5.
6. Lubeck DP, Spitz PW, Fries JF, et al. A multicenter study of annual health service utilization and costs in rheumatoid arthritis. Arthritis Rheum 1986;29:488–93.
7. Wolfe F, Zwillich SH. The long-term outcomes of rheumatoid arthritis: a 23-year prospective, longitudinal study of total joint replacement and its predictors in 1,600 patients with rheumatoid arthritis. Arthritis Rheum 1998;41:1072–82.
8. Wolfe F, Kleinheksel SM, Cathey MA, et al. The clinical value of the Stanford health assessment questionnaire functional disability index in patients with rheumatoid arthritis. J Rheumatol 1988;15:1480–8.
9. Leigh JP, Fries JF. Mortality predictors among 263 patients with rheumatoid arthritis. J Rheumatol 1991;18:1307–12.
10. Pincus T, Brooks RH, Callahan LF. Prediction of long-term mortality in patients with rheumatoid arthritis according to simple questionnaire and joint count measures. Ann Intern Med 1994;120:26–34.
11. Callahan LF, Cordray DS, Wells G, et al. Formal education and five-year mortality in rheumatoid arthritis: mediation by helplessness scale scores. Arthritis Care Res 1996;9:463–72.
12. Callahan LF, Pincus T, Huston JW III, et al. Measures of activity and damage in rheumatoid arthritis: depiction of changes and prediction of mortality over five years. Arthritis Care Res 1997;10:381–94.
13. Söderlin MK, Nieminen P, Hakala M. Functional status predicts mortality in a community based rheumatoid arthritis population. J Rheumatol 1998;25:1895–9.
14. Sokka T, Hakkinen A, Krishnan E, et al. Similar prediction of mortality by the health assessment questionnaire in patients with rheumatoid arthritis and the general population. Ann Rheum Dis 2004;63:494–7.
15. Sokka T, Abelson B, Pincus T. Mortality in rheumatoid arthritis: 2008 update. Clin Exp Rheumatol 2008;26:S35–61.
16. Fries JF, Spitz P, Kraines RG, et al. Measurement of patient outcome in arthritis. Arthritis Rheum 1980;23:137–45.
17. Pincus T, Schur PH, Rose JA, et al. Measurement of serum DNA-binding activity in systemic lupus erythematosus. N Engl J Med 1969;281:701–5.
18. Pincus T. Citation classic. [Pincus T, Schur PH, Rose JA, et al. Measurement of serum DNA-binding in activity in systemic lupus erythematosus. New Engl J Med 1969;281:701–5.]. Current Contents–Clin Pract 1983;11:18.
19. Yazici Y, Bergman M, Pincus T. Time to score quantitative rheumatoid arthritis measures: 28-joint count, disease activity score, health assessment

questionnaire (HAQ), multidimensional HAQ (MDHAQ), and routine assessment of patient index data (RAPID) scores. J Rheumatol 2008;35:603–9.

20. Pincus T, Summey JA, Soraci SA Jr, et al. Assessment of patient satisfaction in activities of daily living using a modified Stanford health assessment questionnaire. Arthritis Rheum 1983;26:1346–53.

21. Pincus T, Callahan LF, Vaughn WK. Questionnaire, walking time and button test measures of functional capacity as predictive markers for mortality in rheumatoid arthritis. J Rheumatol 1987;14:240–51.

22. Pincus T, Swearingen C, Wolfe F. Toward a multidimensional health assessment questionnaire (MDHAQ): assessment of advanced activities of daily living and psychological status in the patient friendly health assessment questionnaire format. Arthritis Rheum 1999;42:2220–30.

23. Pincus T, Sokka T, Kautiainen H. Patients seen for standard rheumatoid arthritis care have significantly better articular, radiographic, laboratory, and functional status in 2000 than in 1985. Arthritis Rheum 2005;52:1009–19.

24. Pincus T, Sokka T, Kautiainen H. Further development of a physical function scale on a multidimensional health assessment questionnaire for standard care of patients with rheumatic diseases. J Rheumatol 2005;32:1432–9.

25. Stucki G, Liang MH, Stucki S, et al. A self-administered rheumatoid arthritis disease activity index (RADAI) for epidemiologic research. Arthritis Rheum 1995;38:795–8.

26. Pincus T, Bergman M, Sokka T, et al. Visual analog scales in formats other than a 10 centimeter horizontal line to assess pain and other clinical data. J Rheumatol 2008;35:1550–8.

27. Pincus T, Swearingen CJ, Bergman MJ et al. RAPID3 on an MDHAQ is correlated significantly with activity levels of DAS28 and CDAI, but scored in 5 versus more than 90 seconds. Arthritis Care Res, in press.

28. Pincus T, Swearingen CJ, Bergman M, et al. RAPID3 (routine assessment of patient index data 3), a rheumatoid arthritis index without formal joint counts for routine care: proposed severity categories compared to DAS and CDAI categories. J Rheumatol 2008;35:2136–47.

29. Pincus T, Bergman MJ, Yazici Y, et al. An index of only patient-reported outcome measures, routine assessment of patient index data 3 (RAPID3), in two abatacept clinical trials: similar results to disease activity score (DAS28) and other RAPID indices that include physician-reported measures. Rheumatology (Oxford) 2008;47:345–9.

30. DeWalt DA, Reed GW, Pincus T. Further clues to recognition of patients with fibromyalgia from a simple 2-page patient multidimensional health assessment questionnaire (MDHAQ). Clin Exp Rheumatol 2004;22:453–61.

31. Wolfe F, Cathey MA, Kleinheksel SM. Fibrositis (fibromyalgia) in rheumatoid arthritis. J Rheumatol 1984;11:814–8.

How to Collect an MDHAQ to Provide Rheumatology Vital Signs (Function, Pain, Global Status, and RAPID3 Scores) in the Infrastructure of Rheumatology Care, Including Some Misconceptions Regarding the MDHAQ

Theodore Pincus, MD[a],*, Alyce M. Oliver, MD, PhD[b],
Martin J. Bergman, MD[c]

KEYWORDS

- MDHAQ • Rheumatology • Questionnaires

The multidimensional health assessment questionnaire (MDHAQ)[1,2] includes scores for physical function, pain, and patient global estimate of status (the 3 patient self-report questionnaire measures in the rheumatoid arthritis [RA] core data set[3–5]), and fatigue, exercise, review of systems, and recent medical history. MDHAQ scores for

A version of this article originally appeared in issue 21(4) of *Best Practice & Research: Clinical Rheumatology*.

This research has been supported in part by grants from Bristol-Myers Squibb and Amgen.

[a] Division of Rheumatology, Department of Medicine, NYU Hospital for Joint Diseases, New York University School of Medicine, New York, NY, USA

[b] Section of Rheumatology, Department of Medicine, Medical College of Georgia, Augusta, GA, USA

[c] Rheumatology, Taylor Hospital, Ridley Park, PA, USA

* Corresponding author.

E-mail address: tedpincus@gmail.com (T. Pincus).

0889-857X/09/$ – see front matter © 2009 Elsevier Inc. All rights reserved.

physical function, pain, patient global estimate, and RAPID3 (routine assessment of patient index data)[6,7] may serve as rheumatology vital signs in patients with chronic rheumatic diseases, and possibly all chronic diseases, analogous to pulse and temperature in acute diseases and blood pressure and cholesterol in health maintenance, as patient history information is prominent in rheumatology management. RAPID3 on an MDHAQ can be calculated in 5 to 10 seconds, without a ruler, calculator, computer, or Web site, in contrast to 106 seconds for a clinical disease activity index (CDAI) score and 114 seconds for a disease activity score (DAS28).[8,9]

The MDHAQ can be used to assess, monitor, establish a prognosis, document changes in status and outcomes, and improve the quality of rheumatology care. This article reviews practical strategies (**Table 1**) to collect an MDHAQ/RAPID3 at every visit of every patient with any rheumatic problem, adapted from previous reports, reviews, and editorials.[6,7,10–14]

ORIENT THE STAFF REGARDING THE IMPORTANCE OF THE MDHAQ IN PATIENT CARE

The use of patient questionnaires requires a change in office procedure, which can seem to add complexity and may engender resistance to change. However, the MDHAQ can streamline the flow of information from patient to physician with quantitative data, review of systems, and medical history, which saves time, supports management decisions, and improves documentation.

If office staff members see the rheumatologist reviewing a questionnaire in clinical care, they are likely to respond positively. However, if questionnaires are presented to the patient in an uncaring manner, or their use is explained as for "research," "documentation," "reimbursement," "collaboration with colleagues," or any reason other than better care of the individual patient, staff members (and patients) lose interest and may resent the apparent extra work.

THE MDHAQ SHOULD BE DISTRIBUTED BY THE CLINIC RECEPTIONIST AS PART OF THE OFFICE INFRASTRUCTURE TO EVERY PATIENT WITH ANY DIAGNOSIS AT EVERY VISIT, AS THE MOST EFFICIENT DISTRIBUTION SYSTEM

The best strategy to assure completion of an MDHAQ is for the receptionist to distribute a questionnaire at each visit of each patient on registration for a visit (**Fig. 1**). Many rheumatologists suggest that patient questionnaires should be used only for certain patients, such as those with RA, or at certain intervals, such as every

Table 1	
Strategy for implementation of the MDHAQ in a physician's office	
1.	Orient the staff regarding the importance of the MDHAQ in patient care
2.	The MDHAQ should be distributed by the clinic receptionist as part of the office infrastructure to every patient with any diagnosis at every visit, as the most efficient distribution system
3.	The MDHAQ should be completed by the patient in the waiting area before the visit, rather than in the examination room or after the visit
4.	Let the patient do as much of the work as possible; the health professional should do as little as possible
5.	The clinician should review the MDHAQ with the patient
6.	Flow sheets are desirable

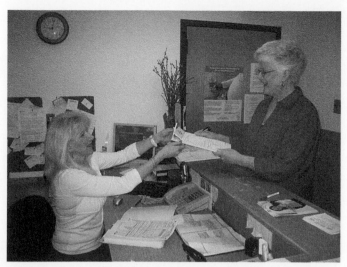

Fig. 1. The best strategy to assure completion of an MDHAQ is for the receptionist to distribute a questionnaire at each visit of each patient on registration for a visit. (*Courtesy of* Dr Martin J. Bergman.)

6 months. This approach generally fails in standard care, as any attempt to distribute questionnaires selectively adds considerably to staff time and complexity. An MDHAQ is useful for all people with all rheumatic diseases (see article 15). If there is a reason for a visit, there is a reason for a questionnaire.

THE MDHAQ SHOULD BE COMPLETED BY THE PATIENT IN THE WAITING AREA BEFORE THE VISIT, RATHER THAN IN THE EXAMINATION ROOM OR AFTER THE VISIT

Most patients spend at least 10 minutes in the waiting room before seeing a rheumatologist, and often longer. This is the time period in which it is most feasible and desirable for a patient to complete a questionnaire (**Fig. 2**). Completion before the encounter helps to focus patient concerns to prepare for the visit. Availability of the data to the physician at the time of the visit is helpful, analogous to availability of a radiograph to an orthopedist at the time a patient is seen, particularly in view of the importance of information from the patient in clinical decisions in rheumatic diseases (in contrast to many chronic diseases). It may seem attractive to mail a questionnaire to the patient to be completed before the visit. This practice is undesirable as responses may differ at the time of the visit, and the patient may forget to bring the questionnaire. An office that functions efficiently so that patients usually wait less than 10 minutes to see the physician can schedule patients 10 minutes earlier to include time for completion of an MDHAQ.

LET THE PATIENT DO AS MUCH OF THE WORK AS POSSIBLE; THE HEALTH PROFESSIONAL SHOULD DO AS LITTLE AS POSSIBLE

Health professionals have substantially more knowledge than the patient concerning disease pathogenesis, treatments, and outcomes, and may feel more qualified to complete a questionnaire than the patient herself or himself. Indeed, certain information that the patient may report, such as diagnosis and comorbidities, seems to be most accurately recorded by a health professional.[15] However, the patient has

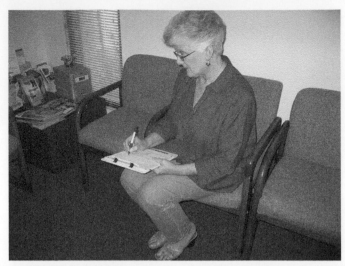

Fig. 2. The MDHAQ should be completed by the patient in the waiting area before the visit, rather than in the examination room or after the visit. Completion before the encounter helps to focus patient concerns to prepare for the visit, particularly in view of the importance of information from the patient in clinical decisions in rheumatic diseases (in contrast to many chronic diseases). (*Courtesy of* Dr Martin J. Bergman.)

superior knowledge to a health professional (or anyone else) concerning most items on the MDHAQ or other validated patient questionnaire, including capacity to perform activities, pain, fatigue, and global estimate of status.

When a patient completes the questionnaire without any input from a health professional (or family member, or anyone else), only 1 observer is involved. Any input from a health professional introduces a second observer, which has been found to reduce accuracy and reproducibility.[16] The health professional may interject a tone from which the patient takes a cue, leading to tendencies to express better or poorer status based on these cues. Therefore, health professionals should avoid, as much as possible, participation in completion of a patient self-report questionnaire, and allow patients to complete the questionnaire with minimal assistance.

If a patient asks "How should I answer a question?" or "I have pain, but not caused by my arthritis" (eg, back pain or recent fracture in a patient with RA), the response of the health professional should be "The answer is whatever you say. There are no right or wrong answers." The patient will provide a baseline and serve as the "gold standard" against which to monitor changes in status. It may be difficult for some health professionals to refrain from becoming involved in the process, but such restraint ensures the most reliable data.

Some patients may need help; for example, an illiterate patient, or one with a language barrier. Many such patients have a literacy or language partner to help them in the clinical setting. The partner is usually preferable to the health professional for helping the patient, as this person is likely to be consistent from visit to visit. Nonetheless, in some situations, help from a health professional is required. Data on a patient self-report questionnaire completed with assistance of a health professional are preferable to no data at all. However, the health professional should do everything possible to be neutral, allowing the patient whatever she or he regards as an appropriate response.

THE CLINICIAN SHOULD REVIEW THE MDHAQ WITH THE PATIENT

Review of the MDHAQ by the physician with the patient (**Fig. 3**) is essential to the success of questionnaire completion in the infrastructure of usual care. Such a review improves the quality and efficiency of a patient visit. The 5 to 10 seconds involved provide information that often would require 2 to 5 minutes of query, particularly the recent medical history, and greater efficiency is inevitable.

It should be emphasized that lack of interest on the part of the physician leads to resistance of staff and patients and is the primary reason for failure of implementation of questionnaire completion at most settings. In the clinical care of the senior author, every patient has completed an HAQ or MDHAQ at every visit since 1982. The mean educational level in Tennessee (and in that clinic population) is lower than the United States median.

If the patient is in the examination room but has not completed the questionnaire, the physician says, "I'll be back in 5 minutes, so I can review your questionnaire scores to help me see how you're doing, and to help us decide how best to treat you." To fill the time, the physician can always find an activity that requires 5 minutes, such as returning a telephone call or reviewing correspondence. This practice establishes the importance of the questionnaire to patients and staff, but is rarely necessary.

FLOW SHEETS ARE DESIRABLE

Convenient entry onto a flow sheet (**Fig. 4**), along with laboratory tests and medications, organizes information to track scores serially on 1 page (see article 16). This information provides an overview at a glance of the patient's course, which is a cost-effective procedure. The senior author produces an electronically generated flow sheet from a Microsoft Access database on each patient at each visit, which includes MDHAQ scores, laboratory tests, and medications, to be available at the

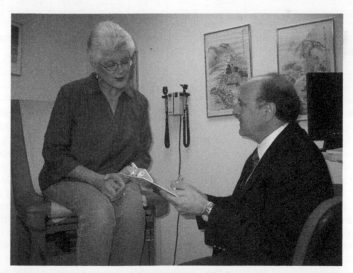

Fig. 3. The review by the physician of the MDHAQ with the patient improves the quality and efficiency of a patient visit. The 5 to 10 seconds for such a review, particularly the recent medical history, provides information that would often involve 2 to 5 minutes of query, and greater efficiency is inevitable. (*Courtesy of* Dr Martin J. Bergman.)

COMPLETED FLOWSHEET: 61 year old male with RA

PT Name_____ DX ICD9___710.9_____, Onset(mo/yr)____ Record#_____

Rheumatologist_____, 1st Visit(mo/yr) 4Nov03, RF: Pos / Neg If+,titer_____, ANA: Pos / Neg If+,titer___

Address_____City, ST ZIP_____Home tel_____

SSN#_____, DOB_____, Sex M / F , Marital Status: _____, Race:_____

Work st:_____, Occ:_____#Yrs Educ____, Consent given: Y / N, 1° MD_____MD Tel_____

DATE	4Nov03	13Jan04	20Jul04	28ep04	28Dec04	08Feb05	28Mar06
M FUNCTIONAL STATUS (FN) [0-10]	3.3	0	0	0	0	0	0
D PAIN (PN) [0-10]	9.5	0.5	3.5	0.5	6.0	0	0.5
H PATIENT GLOBAL (PTGL) [0-10]	9.5	0.5	2.0	1.0	5.5	0	0.5
A RAPID 3 [0-30]	22.3	1.0	5.5	1.5	11.5/4.0	0/0	1.0/0.3
Q PT JOINT COUNT (JT CT) [0-10]					1.9	0	0
RAPID 4 [0-40]					13.4/3.5	0/0	1.0/0.3
PHYSICIAN GLOBAL (MDACT) [0-10]					6.5	1.0	0.5
RAPID 5 [0-50]					19.9/4.0	1.0/0.2	1.5/0.4
WEIGHT (lbs)	167	167	163.8	159	168	166	171
BLOOD PRESSURE (mm/Hg)	114/70	131/81	116/76	128/80	111/71	120/72	129/79
L ESR (mm/hr) [M:0-20 / F:0-30]	43	8	11	10	14	14	14
A CRP (mg/dL) [0-10]	30	3		7	6	8	9.3
B WBC (thou/uL) [4-11]	6.3	7.9	7.1	8.1	9.1	9.6	9.4
O HGB(g/dL-M:14/F:12] OR HCT(%)[M:42/ F:37]	16.8	17	15.9	16.1	16.6	17	15.3
R PLATELETS (thou/uL) [150-400]	179	207	184	203	207	177	193
A ALBUMIN (g/dL) [3.5-5.0]	3.9	4.1	4.4	4	4.4	4.6	4.1
T SGOT (U/L) [4-40] OR SGPT (U/L) [4-40]	18	17	22	18	20	32	21
O CREATININE (mg/dL) [0.7-1.5]	1.1	0.8	0.9	0.9	0.9	1.1	1.0
R							
Y							

MED CODES: N- new drug, O-on at visit, X-toxicity, C-change dose, D-discontinue, T-taper, R-resume, I-injection, V-only today

Naproxen	O-880 Q6H	440 BID	440 BID	440 BID	440 BID	D-440 BID	
M Ranitidine	O-150 BID	150 BID	150 BID	150 BID	150 BID	150 BID	75 BID
E **D** Acetaminophen with Codeine	O-30 TID	30 TID	D-30 TID				
I Prednisone	N-3 QD	1 BID	C-4 BID	C-3 BID	T-3 BID	T-2 BID	C-5 QD
C **A** Methotrexate	N-10 QWK	20 QWK	C-15 QWK	15 QWK	C-25 QWK	15 QWK	15 QWK
T Folic Acid	N-1 QD	1 QD	1 QD	1 QD	1 QD	1 QD	1 QD
I **O** Adalimumab					N-40 QOW	40 QOW	40 QOW
N **S** Depo-Medrol					V-80		

Fig. 4. Flow sheet to facilitate longitudinal assessment of patient in usual rheumatology clinical care. The flow sheet shown is of a man who presented at age 61 with RA. He presented on November 4, 2003 with scores for physical function of 3.3, pain 9.5, global status 9.5, and a RAPID3 score of 22.3 (on a scale of 0–30). He was treated with methotrexate 10 mg/wk and prednisone 3 mg/d. Two months later, on January 13, 2004, his RAPID3 score was 1, indicating a near-remission. He did well for almost a year, as documented for visits on July 20 and September 28, 2004 (his RAPID3 score was 5.5 on July 20, but this was caused by acute back strain and not inflammation, so his therapy was not altered). On December 28, 2004 he presented with a severe flare. His joints were once again swollen, and although his physical function score was 0, his pain was 6.0 and global 5.5. He was offered the possibility of an anti-tumor necrosis factor agent, adalimumab, which he elected to receive. Two months later, on February 5, 2005, all his scores were 0, indicating an excellent response. This status was maintained for more than a year, as indicated by his visit of March 28, 2006.

next visit. However, it is not necessary to use a computer (pencil and paper were used effectively in the 1980s) although computerization is increasing with the growth of electronic medical records (EMRs). Computerization is necessary for analyses and reports of patients in groups. Nonetheless, automation of data should be pursued to the level of comfort of the rheumatologist and staff.

Several reports have reviewed reasons expressed by physicians for not using patient questionnaires.[17,18] Some of the listed reasons, and further concerns stated by rheumatologists, are presented in **Table 2**, and the following sections give explanations of why these are misconceptions.

"I CAN TELL WHETHER MY PATIENT IS DOING WELL OR NOT WITHOUT AN MDHAQ OR RAPID3 SCORE"

The treating clinician and patient have a sense of the patient's clinical status and change from a previous visit. It has been emphasized in many articles in this issue that patient history data are more prominent in clinical management of rheumatic diseases than in many other types of diseases. For example, when a patient sees a physician for management of hypertension, hyperlipidemia, osteoporosis, or many other conditions, the patient must learn from the doctor how well the condition is controlled, rather than informing the doctor.

At the same time, expressing (and recording) status quantitatively adds considerable accuracy that is not available from a mere description. For example, suggesting that a fever is "improved" or even "resolved" is not so informative as noting that it has changed from 104°F to 101°F, or to 98.6°F (or from 40°C to 38°C, or to 37°C). Perhaps even more importantly, quantitative data are needed to document improvement (or worsening) to a third party, whether it is another physician or a payer. Patient

Table 2
Misperceptions frequently expressed as reasons for not using patient self-report questionnaires in usual clinical care
1. "I can tell whether my patient is doing well or not without an MDHAQ or RAPID3 score"
2. "Patient questionnaires add extra time and interfere with patient flow"
3. "Many patients object to completing a questionnaire"
4. "How can I monitor a patient who has RA quantitatively without a formal joint count?"
5. "Patient questionnaire scores are influenced by irreversible damage, unlike joint counts, so they are not so sensitive to control of inflammation"
6. "Patient questionnaire data do not give me so good information to guide clinical decisions and prognosis as traditional radiographic or laboratory measures"
7. "RAPID3 scores may be increased in patients who have fibromyalgia and do not have an inflammatory disease"
8. "The MDHAQ is useful only in RA and not in other rheumatic diseases"
9. "Does a patient questionnaire not eliminate the need to examine patients?"
10. "Does a patient questionnaire not replace conversation and interfere with doctor-patient communication?"
11. "MDHAQ and RAPID3 responses are used to trigger automatic therapeutic decisions"
12. "Patient questionnaire should be used only at certain intervals rather than at each visit"
13. "Electronic data capture is invariably more effective than pencil and paper"
14. "An MDHAQ cannot be completed by patients of low educational level"

testimonials suggest that rheumatologists help their patients as much as any other type of doctor, but without quantitative data it is not possible to document this phenomenon.

"PATIENT QUESTIONNAIRES ADD EXTRA TIME AND INTERFERE WITH PATIENT FLOW"

Completion of an MDHAQ by each patient in usual clinical care adds almost no burden to patient flow, if the questionnaire is distributed when the patient registers for the visit, and is completed by the patient in the waiting room before being seen in the examination room. Scoring of a RAPID3 adds 5 to 10 seconds, which can be accomplished by a receptionist, office assistant, nurse, or physician. The review of systems and recent medical history on the MDHAQ saves time for the patient and physician, and improves documentation.

"MANY PATIENTS OBJECT TO COMPLETING A QUESTIONNAIRE"

Many people initially do not like to be asked to do anything that they have not done previously, such as asking a receptionist to present a questionnaire or asking a patient to complete the questionnaire in the waiting area. Furthermore, if the staff project an attitude that this is a "necessary evil" or "for research" or "to document for insurance," and the physician does not review the questionnaire with the patient, everyone will lose interest. However, staff and patients are responsive to the physician. If the physician reviews the questionnaire with each patient, patients quickly understand that this is an important component of their medical care.

Patient history data are more prominent in rheumatology management decisions than in many other diseases. Many patients say that they find the experience of completing a questionnaire useful for focusing on the encounter; attention to a questionnaire often seems preferable to reading irrelevant material in the waiting room. It is unusual, in settings in which questionnaires are used routinely, for the patient to say at the end of the visit, "Oh, Doctor, I forgot to tell you…", which is not uncommon in usual care settings.

A few patients may object to completing a questionnaire, just as some patients are unwilling to have blood tests or radiographs. The patient's wishes should always be accommodated. Nonetheless, almost all patients do not object and may recognize the questionnaire as helpful for their medical care.

"HOW CAN I MONITOR A PATIENT WHO HAS RA QUANTITATIVELY WITHOUT A FORMAL JOINT COUNT?"

A formal joint count is the most specific measure to assess inflammation in patients with RA. However, the formal joint count has several limitations (see article 3). The greater specificity of a measure does not necessarily indicate greater sensitivity to change, compared with a less-specific measure. Relative efficiencies of all core data set measures to distinguish active from control treatments in clinical trials are similar.[7,19]

"PATIENT QUESTIONNAIRE SCORES ARE INFLUENCED BY IRREVERSIBLE DAMAGE, UNLIKE JOINT COUNTS, SO THEY ARE NOT SO SENSITIVE TO CONTROL OF INFLAMMATION"

Patient questionnaire scores may reflect "irreversible" changes, analogous to radiographs, which might compromise their sensitivity to change with treatment.[20] However, it seems that joint counts also may be influenced by irreversible changes, as the relative efficiencies of all core data set measures to distinguish active from control treatments in clinical trials are similar, as noted earlier.[7,19] Questionnaire scores, although affected by irreversible changes, vary as much as joint counts or C-reactive protein levels in short and long periods to document control, or absence of control, of inflammation.

"PATIENT QUESTIONNAIRE DATA DO NOT GIVE ME SO GOOD INFORMATION TO GUIDE CLINICAL DECISIONS AND PROGNOSIS AS TRADITIONAL RADIOGRAPHIC OR LABORATORY MEASURES"

The traditional biomedical model, the dominant paradigm of twentieth-century medicine,[21,22] values laboratory tests and radiographs as considerably more informative than patient questionnaires. However, patient-derived information is usually more prominent in clinical decisions than laboratory tests and radiographs in rheumatic diseases, compared with most other diseases. Patient questionnaires also are more significant to predict long-term work disability, costs, and premature mortality than laboratory tests or radiographs.[23] Therefore, the patient questionnaire can be as useful as any measure in clinical care. Furthermore, patient questionnaires are less expensive than other measures.

"RAPID3 SCORES MAY BE INCREASED IN PATIENTS WHO HAVE FIBROMYALGIA AND DO NOT HAVE AN INFLAMMATORY DISEASE"

It is recognized that RAPID3 scores may be increased in patients who have fibromyalgia (see article 20). These patients usually have scores for pain and global estimate of status greater than 6 (on a scale of 0–10), which alone would put them in the category of high severity, with RAPID3 score greater than 12 (see article 9). As noted earlier, it has never been suggested that RAPID3 scores alone should be used for diagnosis and management in the absence of further history, physical examination, laboratory tests, and imaging studies.

All measures in rheumatology (or clinical medicine in general) require interpretation. Even the DAS28 may be increased to a level of apparent "high activity," even in the absence of any swollen joints. For example, a patient who has a tender joint count of 28, swollen joint count of 0, erythrocyte sedimentation rate (ESR) of 20, and global estimate of 6 would have a DAS28 of 5.12 (http://www.das-score.nl/www.das-score.nl/dasculators.html), which would be interpreted as "high activity" (see article 7).

The DAS is not performed in patients with fibromyalgia in the absence of RA. However, RAPID3 should be interpreted with inclusion of all other data concerning the patient. Furthermore, analysis of RAPID3 components, that is, the ratio of pain to physical function scores, can be a clue to fibromyalgia (see article 20).[24,25]

"THE MDHAQ IS USEFUL ONLY IN RA AND NOT IN OTHER RHEUMATIC DISEASES"

Most patients who see a rheumatologist are likely to have problems concerning physical function, pain, global estimate of status, and fatigue (see article 15). Scores for these problems are regarded as "rheumatology vital signs," of which all physicians should be aware (see article 10). All patients require a review of systems and recent medical history, which are available to the physician from the MDHAQ. The MDHAQ is useful in patients with all rheumatic diseases.[12]

"DOES A PATIENT QUESTIONNAIRE NOT ELIMINATE THE NEED TO EXAMINE PATIENTS?"

A patient questionnaire is an adjunct to care, just like a radiograph or laboratory test. It has been suggested that a formal quantitative joint count may not be necessary, as a patient questionnaire provides quantitative data of similar value to monitor patients (see article 3). However, all visits of patients to a rheumatologist must include a careful further history and physical examination, including a careful joint examination, and laboratory tests and radiographs in many situations, for optimal interpretation of MDHAQ and RAPID3 scores.

"DOES A PATIENT QUESTIONNAIRE NOT REPLACE CONVERSATION AND INTERFERE WITH DOCTOR-PATIENT COMMUNICATION?"

The patient questionnaire not only does not interfere with doctor-patient communication but it adds to it by directing the discussion to address patient concerns more directly. A careful history is always needed for diagnosis and management, and a patient questionnaire can provide factual information to save time for the doctor and patient.

Many patients with RA have such good clinical status that they do not require lengthy visits, but nonetheless require careful monitoring of therapy with methotrexate or biologic agents. Some of these patients are anxious to return to work, and do not necessarily require a lengthy visit with extensive conversation. These patients can be accommodated using the patient questionnaire to add appropriate documentation of efficient care.

"MDHAQ AND RAPID3 RESPONSES ARE USED TO TRIGGER AUTOMATIC THERAPEUTIC DECISIONS"

The introduction of quantitative measures into clinical rheumatology may suggest essentially "automatic" responses, such as "anyone with a high RAPID3 score greater than 12, or a DAS28 greater than 5.1, or a CDAI score more than 22 must have a change in disease-modifying antirheumatic drug (DMARD) or biologic therapy." A change in therapy should certainly be considered for patients with these values. However, RAPID3 or any measure should serve only as a guide to clinical judgment, although clinical judgment is greatly enhanced by availability of quantitative measures.

For example, a patient may have an increased ESR or DAS28 compared with a previous visit, which may reflect infection or development of a lymphoma, rather than a flare of RA. A history and physical examination, and other laboratory tests, are required to understand the basis for a change in a quantitative measure. Similarly, a patient may sustain a compression fracture, raising global scores, and thereby raising RAPID3, DAS28, or CDAI scores, but not require a change in therapy.

"PATIENT QUESTIONNAIRES SHOULD BE USED ONLY AT CERTAIN INTERVALS RATHER THAN AT EACH VISIT"

Some rheumatologists suggest that they would like to administer the questionnaire only to people with RA, or only every 3 months. Such approaches generally fail, for several reasons. Asking the receptionist to recognize whether or not a patient should be given a questionnaire adds complexity, resulting in complaints from the staff, and a view of the questionnaire as a burden rather than a routine matter. Furthermore, the diagnosis is unknown in new patients (and sometimes in returning patients). Long-term studies indicate that, among patients with any specific rheumatologic diagnosis who are monitored for a decade or longer, at least a few have a change in diagnosis.

The most efficient method to use the MDHAQ in usual care is for the receptionist to distribute the questionnaire to every patient at every visit. Most patients are seen in rheumatology clinical settings every 2 to 6 months, although a patient with an unusual condition may be seen every 1 or 2 weeks. If there is a reason for a patient to be seen frequently, there is even more of a reason to assess clinical status quantitatively, to recognize improvement or worsening of clinical status.

"ELECTRONIC DATA CAPTURE IS INVARIABLY MORE EFFECTIVE THAN PENCIL AND PAPER"

Many suggest it is desirable for the patient to enter response data directly into an electronic database, to provide an accurate score. Direct entry into a computer eliminates the need for someone else to enter it into a database. However, programing and maintenance of computers for direct entry often add to costs, which may then be greater than costs of simple data entry. Furthermore, direct entry by patients seems too complex in most clinical settings, other than in specialized clinics with sophisticated computer systems.

A physician cannot open a computer file and calculate a RAPID3 score more quickly than in 5 to 10 seconds. In general, pencil and paper are more efficient and less costly than direct entry by the patient on a computer. An EMR is not an electronic database (see article 16). One should be careful about the overuse of technology; many attractive options are expensive and based on "hotel-based medicine"[26] rather than actual clinical care.

"AN MDHAQ CANNOT BE COMPLETED BY PATIENTS OF LOW EDUCATIONAL LEVEL"

About 20% of patients of low educational levels experience difficulty with completion of a questionnaire.[27] Furthermore, patients of low educational levels generally have poorer status according to the MDHAQ and also have poorer status according to joint counts and ESR, reflecting poorer overall clinical status of patients with lower socioeconomic status.[28] Illiterate patients may receive some help from a family member, but generally have a literacy partner to help them reach the clinic and function in society in general.[29] An MDHAQ has been recorded on every patient seen at every visit since 1980 in the senior author's clinical care, regardless of socioeconomic status (or any other variable), in Tennessee, where educational level and literacy are lower than the median for the United States.

SUMMARY

The MDHAQ is easily completed by patients, and a RAPID3 score gives results that are similar to the widely recognized indices DAS28 and CDAI, in less than 10% of the time. Simple strategies are available for distribution, collection, and management of the MDHAQ and RAPID3.[14] It has been proposed that "80% of the data in 100% of the patients may be preferable to 100% of the data in 5% of the patients" (or fewer) who might be included in clinical research.[30] An MDHAQ and RAPID3 score may provide "80% of the data in 100% of patients," particularly in view of the importance of patient information in rheumatology clinical decisions. Even if less specific or comprehensive, an MDHAQ that is feasible and applicable in usual clinical care seems preferable to no quantitative measure at all.

The MDHAQ and RAPID3 scores provide informative quantitative data for patient status from 1 visit to the next. If quantitative data are recorded, an opportunity for documentation and more rational monitoring is gained, along with enhanced efficiency of patient care. If no data are recorded, this opportunity is lost and can never be replaced.

It is suggested that all rheumatologists would find it valuable to ask all patients to complete an MDHAQ, and to score a RAPID3 (themselves or by a staff member), at all visits of all patients in usual care. Use of MDHAQ/RAPID3 by all rheumatologists could transform clinical rheumatology from a descriptive field (apart from clinical trials and other clinical research studies), so that all care can be conducted in quantitative rather than descriptive terms. Clinical rheumatology could then have a firmer scientific basis, with accurate assessment of patient status at each visit, better guidance for clinical monitoring, better patient outcomes, and increased respect as a quantitative science. Nonetheless, all quantitative measures, ranging from hemoglobin to ESR to RAPID3, must be viewed in the context of all data from the individual patient in formulating clinical decisions. All medical care must be tailored to each individual patient; global recommendations, including levels of RA indices that may suggest changes in therapy, must be viewed as guidelines, and not as absolute directives.

REFERENCES

1. Pincus T, Swearingen C, Wolfe F. Toward a multidimensional health assessment questionnaire (MDHAQ): assessment of advanced activities of daily living and psychological status in the patient friendly health assessment questionnaire format. Arthritis Rheum 1999;42:2220–30.
2. Pincus T, Sokka T, Kautiainen H. Further development of a physical function scale on a multidimensional health assessment questionnaire for standard care of patients with rheumatic diseases. J Rheumatol 2005;32:1432–9.
3. Felson DT, Anderson JJ, Boers M, et al. The American College of Rheumatology preliminary core set of disease activity measures for rheumatoid arthritis clinical trials. Arthritis Rheum 1993;36:729–40.
4. Tugwell P, Boers M. OMERACT Committee. Proceedings of the OMERACT conferences on outcome measures in rheumatoid arthritis clinical trials, Maastricht, Netherlands. J Rheumatol 1993;20:527–91.
5. Boers M, Tugwell P, Felson DT, et al. World Health Organization and International League of Associations for Rheumatology core endpoints for symptom modifying antirheumatic drugs in rheumatoid arthritis clinical trials. J Rheumatol 1994; 21(Suppl 41):86–9.
6. Pincus T, Yazici Y, Bergman M, et al. A proposed continuous quality improvement approach to assessment and management of patients with rheumatoid arthritis without formal joint counts, based on quantitative routine assessment of patient index data (RAPID) scores on a multidimensional health assessment questionnaire (MDHAQ). Best Pract Res Clin Rheumatol 2007;21:789–804.
7. Pincus T, Bergman MJ, Yazici Y, et al. An index of only patient-reported outcome measures, routine assessment of patient index data 3 (RAPID3), in two abatacept clinical trials: similar results to disease activity score (DAS28) and other RAPID indices that include physician-reported measures. Rheumatology (Oxford) 2008;47:345–9.
8. Yazici Y, Bergman M, Pincus T. Time to score quantitative rheumatoid arthritis measures: 28-joint count, disease activity score, health assessment questionnaire (HAQ), multidimensional HAQ (MDHAQ), and routine assessment of patient index data (RAPID) scores. J Rheumatol 2008;35:603–9.

9. Pincus T, Swearingen CJ, Bergman MJ, et al. RAPID3 on an MDHAQ is correlated significantly with activity levels of DAS28 and CDAI, but scored in 5 versus more than 90 seconds. Arthritis Care Res, in press.
10. Pincus T, Yazici Y, Bergman M, et al. A proposed approach to recognize "near-remission" quantitatively without formal joint counts or laboratory tests: a patient self-report questionnaire routine assessment of patient index data (RAPID) score as a guide to a "continuous quality improvement" strategy. Clin Exp Rheumatol 2006;24(6 Suppl 43):S60–5.
11. Pincus T, Yazici Y, Bergman M. A practical guide to scoring a multi-dimensional health assessment questionnaire (MDHAQ) and routine assessment of patient index data (RAPID) scores in 10–20 seconds for use in standard clinical care, without rulers, calculators, websites or computers. Best Pract Res Clin Rheumatol 2007;21:755–87.
12. Pincus T, Sokka T. Can a multi-dimensional health assessment questionnaire (MDHAQ) and routine assessment of patient index data (RAPID) scores be informative in patients with all rheumatic diseases? Best Pract Res Clin Rheumatol 2007;21:733–53.
13. Pincus T, Yazici Y, Bergman M. Saving time and improving care with a multidimensional health assessment questionnaire: 10 practical considerations. J Rheumatol 2006;33:448–54.
14. Pincus T. Pain, function, and RAPID scores - vital signs in chronic diseases, analogous to pulse and temperature in acute diseases and blood pressure and cholesterol in long-term health. Bull NYU Hosp Jt Dis 2008;66:155–65.
15. Kvien TK, Glennås A, Knudsrod OG, et al. The validity of self-reported diagnosis of rheumatoid arthritis: results from a population survey followed by clinical examinations. J Rheumatol 1996;23:1866–71.
16. Fries JF, Spitz P, Kraines RG, et al. Measurement of patient outcome in arthritis. Arthritis Rheum 1980;23:137–45.
17. Wolfe F, Pincus T, Thompson AK, et al. The assessment of rheumatoid arthritis and the acceptability of self-report questionnaires in clinical practice. Arthritis Care Res 2003;49:59–63.
18. Russak SM, Croft JD Jr, Furst DE, et al. The use of rheumatoid arthritis health-related quality of life patient questionnaire in clinical practice: lessons learned. Arthritis Rheum 2003;49:574–84.
19. Strand V, Cohen S, Crawford B, et al. Patient-reported outcomes better discriminate active treatment from placebo in randomized controlled trials in rheumatoid arthritis. Rheumatology 2004;43:640–7.
20. Aletaha D, Smolen J, Ward MM. Measuring function in rheumatoid arthritis: identifying reversible and irreversible components. Arthritis Rheum 2006;54:2784–92.
21. Engel GL. The need for a new medical model: a challenge for biomedicine. Science 1977;196:129–36.
22. Callahan LF, Pincus T. Education, self-care, and outcomes of rheumatic diseases: further challenges to the "biomedical model" paradigm. Arthritis Care Res 1997;10:283–8.
23. Pincus T. Clinical observations often provide more accurate information concerning the long-term natural history and results of treatment for rheumatoid arthritis than structured research studies. Rheumatol Eur 1995;24:179–84.
24. Callahan LF, Pincus T. The P-VAS/D-ADL ratio: a clue from a self-report questionnaire to distinguish rheumatoid arthritis from noninflammatory diffuse musculoskeletal pain. Arthritis Rheum 1990;33:1317–22.

25. DeWalt DA, Reed GW, Pincus T. Further clues to recognition of patients with fibromyalgia from a simple 2-page patient multidimensional health assessment questionnaire (MDHAQ). Clin Exp Rheumatol 2004;22:453–61.
26. Pincus T, Yazici Y, Bergman MJ. Hotel-based medicine. J Rheumatol 2008;35: 1487–8.
27. Callahan LF, Brooks RH, Summey JA, et al. Quantitative pain assessment for routine care of rheumatoid arthritis patients, using a pain scale based on activities of daily living and a visual analogue pain scale. Arthritis Rheum 1987;30: 630–6.
28. Callahan LF, Pincus T. Formal education level as a significant marker of clinical status in rheumatoid arthritis. Arthritis Rheum 1988;31:1346–57.
29. DeWalt DA, Berkman ND, Sheridan S, et al. Literacy and health outcomes: a systematic review of the literature. J Gen Intern Med 2004;19:1228–39.
30. Pincus T, Wolfe F. Patient questionnaires for clinical research and improved standard patient care: is it better to have 80% of the information in 100% of patients or 100% of the information in 5% of patients? J Rheumatol 2005;32:575–7.

Quantitative Recording of Physician Clinical Estimates, Beyond a Global Estimate and Formal Joint Count, in Usual Care: Applying the Scientific Method, Using a Simple One-Page Worksheet

Theodore Pincus, MD[a],*, Martin J. Bergman, MD[b]

KEYWORDS

- Physician global estimate • Damage estimate
- Prognosis estimate • Fibromyalgia/somatization estimate

Patient self-report questionnaires may be regarded as a standardized, quantitative, scientific format of a patient history. The prominence of patient information in clinical management of rheumatic diseases renders patient questionnaires quite important. Nonetheless, there remains a need for information from a further medical history, physical examination, laboratory tests, and imaging studies to guide optimal clinical decisions.

A version of this article originally appeared in the 21:4 issue of *Best Practice & Research: Clinical Rheumatology*.

[a] Division of Rheumatology, Department of Medicine, New York University School of Medicine and NYU Hospital for Joint Diseases, 301 East 17th Street, Room 1608, New York, NY 10003, USA

[b] Rheumatology, Taylor Hospital, Ridley Park, PA, USA

* Corresponding author.

E-mail address: tedpincus@gmail.com (T. Pincus).

It is curious that over the last 30 years, in rheumatology, extensive attention has been directed to quantitation of clinical data reported by the patient, but little attention to quantitation of data from the physician. A minority of rheumatologists perform a standard formal quantitative joint count,[1,2] outside of clinical trials and other clinical research,[3] although a careful nonquantitative joint examination generally is performed. The only quantitative measures available at most regular rheumatology encounters are laboratory tests, which frequently are not available at the time of the visit and may be uninformative in many patients. It would appear of value for a physician to record a minimum set of quantitative estimates at a rheumatology visits, which appear of value to establish a prognosis and rationale for clinical decisions.

The corresponding author has used a simple, one-page worksheet since 1995 to record certain basic information concerning each patient seen at each visit (**Fig. 1**). The worksheet includes a physician global estimate of status on a 0 to 10 visual analog scale (VAS) and estimate of change in status on a 0 to 10 VAS, with "no change" being a score of 5. Six simple scales are completed by circling a 0 to 3 scale (0 = none, 1 = low, 2 = moderate, 3 = high) for: (1) degree of inflammation at any time, (2) degree of inflammation at the time of the visit, (3) degree of organ damage, (4) degree of fibromyalgia or somatization, (5) estimated prognosis with no therapy, and (6) estimated prognosis with available therapies. All changes in medications—discontinuations, new starts, change in dosage—are recorded. A template is available for a formal 42-joint count, including the number of swollen joints, tender joints, joints with deformity or limited motion, joints with surgery, and a space to indicate a joint with none of these abnormalities. This worksheet is described in greater detail below.

The first item recorded is the physician global estimate VAS, which has the highest relative efficiency of all rheumatoid arthritis (RA) Core Data Set measures[4] to distinguish active from control treatment in four adalimumab clinical trials,[5] and generally higher relative efficiency than tender and swollen joint counts in clinical trials of methotrexate,[6,7] leflunomide,[6,7] and abatacept.[8] Ironically, the physician global estimate is characterized by the least psychometric analysis of any of the seven RA Core Data Set measures.[5] It has been suggested (Frederick Wolfe, personal communication, 2001) that the physician adjusts for all types of information that is not necessarily found on specific questionnaires or other queries, which inevitably cannot include all important information in management decisions.

The "change" scale VAS allows the physician to estimate quantitatively whether the patient appears better, the same, or worse at a specific visit compared to a previous visit. That estimate may be important in decisions about whether not to institute therapy, or change therapies, or maintain current therapies without change. Documentation on a VAS requires less than 2 seconds.

The degree of inflammation is estimated on two 0 to 3 scales: "ever" and "at this visit." A patient with RA, systemic lupus erythematosus, or other inflammatory rheumatic disease may have been affected by substantial inflammation in the past, but have little inflammation at the time of the visit associated with effective treatment. Nonetheless, the patient is not likely to remain in that state if medications are discontinued. Therefore, recording that there is no evidence of inflammation at a visit is not sufficient in a rationale for management decisions, and an estimate of previous levels of inflammation is also recorded.

A 0 to 3 estimate of damage is of value, as a patient may have substantial symptoms that may be due primarily to irreversible joint or other organ damage, rather than to reversible inflammatory arthritis. The patient's symptoms may suggest a possible

R813   RHEUMATOLOGY HEALTH OUTCOME OFFICE MONITORING (Update R752, R782) Page 1 of 1
PATIENT _____ DATE _____ MD_____

DIAGNOSIS: 1. _____ Onset yr: _____ DIAGNOSIS 2. _____ Onset yr: _____

Assessor rating of **PATIENT GLOBAL STATUS** at this time:
EXCELLENT   O O O O O O O O O O O O O O O O O O O O O   VERY POOR
              0 0.5 1.0 1.5 2.0 2.5 3.0 3.5 4.0 4.5 5.0 5.5 6.0 6.5 7.0 7.5 8.0 8.5 9.0 9.5 10

Assessor rating of **CHANGE SINCE LAST VISIT - OR OVER LAST MONTH** for new patients:
MUCH BETTER O O O O O O O O O O O O O O O O O O O O O   MUCH WORSE
              0 0.5 1.0 1.5 2.0 2.5 3.0 3.5 4.0 4.5 5.0 5.5 6.0 6.5 7.0 7.5 8.0 8.5 9.0 9.5 10
                                               ↑
                                             SAME

Four scales below: 0 = none, 1 = low, 2 = moderate, 3 = high

a. Degree of inflammation <u>EVER</u>: 0, 1, 2, 3   b. Degree of inflammation <u>TODAY</u>:   0, 1, 2, 3
c. Degree of joint damage: 0, 1, 2, 3   d. Degree of fibromyalgia/somatization: 0, 1, 2, 3
e. Prognosis <u>WITHOUT</u> Rx: Excellent,   Very Good,   Good,   Fair,   Poor
f. Prognosis <u>WITH</u> Rx: Excellent,   Very Good,   Good,   Fair,   Poor

DRUG CHANGES SINCE LAST VISIT: Circle one: Yes   None   If Yes, please list below:

NEW DRUGS AND DOSAGE:	CHANGE IN DOSAGE:	DISCONTINUATIONS	(BASIS) D/C Codes:
1._____	1._____	1._____	NO Efficacy
2._____	2._____	2._____	TOXicity
3._____	3._____	3._____	LOSS of Efficacy

42 JOINT COUNT - SCORE EACH JOINT AS:"+"or"POSitive"or"ABNormal" versus"–" or"NEGative" or "NORMal"

	If NORMal mark "NL" & go to next joint	Tender or pain on motion	Swollen	Limited motion or deformed	Number of Surgeries§		If NORMal mark "NL" & go to next joint	Tender or pain on motion	Swollen	Limited motion or de-formed	Number of Surgeries§
R-PIP1	___	___	___	___	___	L-PIP1	___	___	___	___	___
R-PIP2	___	___	___	___	___	L-PIP2	___	___	___	___	___
R-PIP3	___	___	___	___	___	L-PIP3	___	___	___	___	___
R-PIP4	___	___	___	___	___	L-PIP4	___	___	___	___	___
R-PIP5	___	___	___	___	___	L-PIP5	___	___	___	___	___
R-MCP1	___	___	___	___	___	L-MCP1	___	___	___	___	___
R-MCP2	___	___	___	___	___	L-MCP2	___	___	___	___	___
R-MCP3	___	___	___	___	___	L-MCP3	___	___	___	___	___
R-MCP4	___	___	___	___	___	L-MCP4	___	___	___	___	___
R-MCP5	___	___	___	___	___	L-MCP5	___	___	___	___	___
R-WRIST	___	___	___	___	___	**L-WRIST**	___	___	___	___	___
R-ELBOW	___	___	___	___	___	**L-ELBOW**	___	___	___	___	___
R-SHLDR	___	___	XXX	___	___	**L-SHLDR**	___	___	XXX	___	___
R-HIP	___	___	XXX	___	___	**L-HIP**	___	___	XXX	___	___
R-KNEE	___	___	___	___	___	**L-KNEE**	___	___	___	___	___
R-ANKLE	___	___	___	___	___	**L-ANKLE**	___	___	___	___	___
R-MTP1	___	___	___	___	___	L-MTP1	___	___	___	___	___
R-MTP2	___	___	___	___	___	L-MTP2	___	___	___	___	___
R-MTP3	___	___	___	___	___	L-MTP3	___	___	___	___	___
R-MTP4	___	___	___	___	___	L-MTP4	___	___	___	___	___
R-MTP5	___	___	___	___	___	L-MTP5	___	___	___	___	___

§ - S = Synovectomy   J = Total Joint Replacement (TJR)   O = Other

Description only - not in formal joint count:

NECK ___ _____   FEET ___ _____
BACK ___ _____   OTHER ___ _____

JOINT COUNT TOTALS: #tender_____   #swollen_____   #deformed/limited motion_____   #surgeries_____

ENCOUNTER JT CT (PART 54, RHOOM137, R234, R362, R367, R380, R492, R549, R573, R752, R782)

Fig. 1. One-page physician data worksheet for standardized recording of patient information at each rheumatology visit. (*From* Health Report Services, Inc; with permission.)

need for more aggressive therapy than is instituted at the visit and a formal estimation of damage may be of value.

A similar rationale underlies recording a 0 to 3 estimate of fibromyalgia-somatization. Patients with fibromyalgia report some of the highest scores on a pain and global status VAS (see "Clues on the MDHAQ to Identify Patients with Fibromyalgia and Similar Chronic Pain Conditions," by Pincus in this issue).[9,10] A recorded quantitative estimate may explain clinical decisions, particularly in the 20% to 30% of patients with RA, systemic lupus erythematosus, or other inflammatory disease whose symptoms arise primarily from fibromyalgia-somatization, or a chronic pain syndrome.[11,12]

Recording of an estimate of prognosis is not regarded as a component of standard medical practice, although this estimate is perhaps the most important composite synthesis of information from a patient history, physical examination, laboratory tests, and imaging studies used by the physician in management decisions. The corresponding author's scale includes five categories: excellent, very good, good, fair, and poor. Two estimates are recorded: one for the patient without therapy, and a second for the patient with available therapies. The second scale is needed because patients with inflammatory rheumatic diseases may have an ominous prognosis, including anticipated premature mortality without therapy, and yet have very good prognosis with therapies that are available at this time.

The worksheet includes recording of all medication changes: new starts, discontinuations, and changes in dosage. Although the standard medical record captures this information, the task of analyzing (1) the likelihood of continuation of a therapy, as was done for methotrexate over 13 years in the corresponding author's clinic,[13] or (2) at what point in the course of disease a new therapy is begun, as has been analyzed for methotrexate over 25 years in the corresponding author's clinic,[14] is greatly simplified by recording of the actual date of initiation and discontinuation of the therapy. It also provides an alert to confirm that it is really the intended treatment plan, which sometimes is useful to confirm the decision, a slight "tickler" asking, ie, "Do you really want to make this change?"

A template is also included for a 42-joint count, which includes the components of the 28-joint count: 10 metacarpal phalangeal joints, 10 proximal interphalangeal joints, wrists, elbows, shoulders, and knees. The 42-joint count also includes hips, ankles, and 10 toes. The findings recorded for each joint include swelling and tenderness, as used in clinical trials, as well as deformity or limited motion to recognize damage. Deformity or limited motion is highly correlated with radiographs, unlike swelling, which is correlated at a lower level; and tenderness, which is not correlated at all with radiographic findings. Also recorded is whether surgery has been performed on the joint and the number of operations, with codes for total joint replacement, synovectomy, or other procedure. A joint might be recorded as "normal" after total joint replacement, which would not necessarily indicate that there is no abnormality. Because four different possible abnormalities can be recorded, a space is available for recording that the joint is entirely normal. This joint count takes about 2 minutes—obviously fewer when there are fewer involved joints.

A version of this worksheet with a homunculus has been requested by several rheumatologists, and is available from the corresponding author. He prefers the list format, which is more amenable to data entry, particularly with four variables recorded, although it recognized that some rheumatologists prefer the homunculus format.

The worksheet is still in an early stage of development—somewhat analogous to patient self-report questionnaires to assess physical function and pain in the 1970s. At the same time, advances in medical care have been greatly facilitated by availability of quantitative data. Completion of this worksheet involves less than 30 seconds without a joint count, and about 2 minutes with a formal joint count. The time spent completing the worksheet and recording the scores in a database could substantially improve clinical care and outcomes. It would appear appropriate that physician impressions, as the basis of clinical decisions, might be recorded in a brief quantitative format to improve care and outcomes.

REFERENCES

1. Decker JL. American Rheumatism Association nomenclature and classification of arthritis and rheumatism. Arthritis Rheum 1983;26:1029–32.
2. Fuchs HA, Brooks RH, Callahan LF, et al. A simplified twenty-eight joint quantitative articular index in rheumatoid arthritis. Arthritis Rheum 1989;32:531–7.
3. Pincus T, Segurado OG. Most visits of most patients with rheumatoid arthritis to most rheumatologists do not include a formal quantitative joint count. Ann Rheum Dis 2006;65:820–2.
4. Felson DT, Anderson JJ, Boers M, et al. The American College of Rheumatology preliminary core set of disease activity measures for rheumatoid arthritis clinical trials. Arthritis Rheum 1993;36:729–40.
5. Pincus T, Amara I, Segurado OG, et al. Relative efficiencies of physician/assessor global estimates and patient questionnaire measures are similar to or greater than joint counts to distinguish adalimumab from control treatments in rheumatoid arthritis clinical trials. J Rheumatol 2008;35:201–5.
6. Strand V, Cohen S, Schiff M, et al. Treatment of active rheumatoid arthritis with leflunomide compared with placebo and methotrexate. Arch Intern Med 1999;159:2542–50.
7. Tugwell P, Wells G, Strand V, et al. Clinical improvement as reflected in measures of function and health-related quality of life following treatment with leflunomide compared with methotrexate in patients with rheumatoid arthritis: sensitivity and relative efficiency to detect a treatment effect in a twelve-month, placebo-controlled trial. Arthritis Rheum 2000;43:506–14.
8. Wells G, Li T, Maxwell L, et al. Responsiveness of patient reported outcomes including fatigue, sleep quality, activity limitation, and quality of life following treatment with abatacept for rheumatoid arthritis. Ann Rheum Dis 2008;67:260–5.
9. Callahan LF, Pincus T. The P-VAS/D-ADL ratio: a clue from a self-report questionnaire to distinguish rheumatoid arthritis from noninflammatory diffuse musculoskeletal pain. Arthritis Rheum 1990;33:1317–22.
10. DeWalt DA, Reed GW, Pincus T. Further clues to recognition of patients with fibromyalgia from a simple 2-page patient multidimensional health assessment questionnaire (MDHAQ). Clin Exp Rheumatol 2004;22:453–61.
11. Wolfe F, Cathey MA, Kleinheksel SM. Fibrositis (fibromyalgia) in rheumatoid arthritis. J Rheumatol 1984;11:814–8.
12. Wolfe F, Petri M, Alarcon GS, et al. Fibromyalgia, systemic lupus erythematosus (SLE), and evaluation of SLE activity. J Rheumatol 2009;36:82–8.
13. Yazici Y, Sokka T, Kautiainen H, et al. Long term safety of methotrexate in routine clinical care: discontinuation is unusual and rarely the result of laboratory abnormalities. Ann Rheum Dis 2005;64:207–11.
14. Sokka T, Pincus T. Ascendancy of weekly low-dose methotrexate in usual care of rheumatoid arthritis from 1980 to 2004 at two sites in Finland and the United States. Rheumatology (Oxford); 2008;47:1543–7.

A Multi-Dimensional Health Assessment Questionnaire (MDHAQ) and Routine Assessment of Patient Index Data (RAPID3) Scores are Informative in Patients with All Rheumatic Diseases

Theodore Pincus, MD[a],*, Anca Dinu Askanase, MD, MPH[a],
Christopher J. Swearingen, PhD[b]

KEYWORDS

- MDHAQ • RAPID3 • Rheumatic diseases
- Quantitative assessment

Rheumatic diseases are not characterized by a single gold standard measure for diagnosis and management of all individual patients. Classification criteria to standardize patient enrollment in clinical research studies that include the four types of measures in a standard medical encounter: patient history, physical examination, laboratory tests, and imaging studies are available for rheumatoid arthritis (RA),[1] ankylosing spondylitis,[2] rheumatic fever,[3] osteoarthritis,[4,5] gout,[6] systemic lupus

---

A version of this article originally appeared in the 21:4 issue of *Best Practice & Research: Clinical Rheumatology*.

Supported in part by grants from the Arthritis Foundation and the Jack Massey Foundation.

[a] Division of Rheumatology, Department of Medicine, New York University School of Medicine and NYU Hospital for Joint Diseases, Room 1608, 301 East 17th Street, New York, NY 10003, USA

[b] Department of Pediatrics, Biostatistics Program, University of Arkansas for Medical Sciences, Little Rock, AR, USA

* Corresponding author.

E-mail address: tedpincus@gmail.com, theodore.pincus@nyumc.org (T. Pincus).

Rheum Dis Clin N Am 35 (2009) 819–827
doi:10.1016/j.rdc.2009.10.017
0889-857X/09/$ – see front matter © 2009 Elsevier Inc. All rights reserved.

erythematosus (SLE),[7,8] systemic sclerosis,[9] polymyositis and dermatomyositis,[10] Sjögren syndrome,[11] vasculitis,[12] Behçet syndrome,[13] and antiphospholipid syndrome,[14] and others. Assessment and monitoring of patient clinical status in rheumatic diseases is described by pooled indices, which also include the tetrad of patient history, physical examination, laboratory tests, and imaging studies. Formal indices have been described for RA,[15-20] SLE,[21-28] vasculitis,[29-34] psoriatic arthritis,[35-37] ankylosing spondylitis,[38-42] and other rheumatic diseases.

Classification criteria and indices to assess status are widely used in clinical research. However, most usual rheumatology care is conducted according to descriptive impressions of the treating rheumatologist, without quantitative measures other than laboratory tests, which often are unavailable at the time of care and give frequent false-positive and false-negative results.[43-45] Therefore, any possible benefits of extensive advances in measurement developed by expert researchers are available to only a very small fraction of patients seen by rheumatologists.

A primary explanation for the absence of quantitative clinical measurement in usual rheumatology care involves the difficulty of collecting and scoring complex measures and indices in busy clinical settings. Measures and indices designed for research differ from measures designed for usual care (see "Complex Measures and Indices for Clinical Research Compared with Simple Patient Questionnaires to Assess Function, Pain, and Global Estimates as Rheumatology "Vital Signs" for Usual Clinical Care," by Pincus T, et al, in this issue). Most rheumatology visits are conducted in fewer than 30 minutes, and attention to patient concerns to formulate a nonquantitative assessment usually presents a higher priority than exact quantitative measurement.

A goal of some quantitative measurement in standard rheumatology care would appear desirable, as quantitative measures have greatly advanced patient care in many domains. Quantitative measures provide more accurate information than available from nonquantitative impressions concerning patient status at baseline and over time, and better documentation and outcomes. Six clinical trials[46-51] document that clinical care guided by a disease activity score (DAS28),[15,16] with target values to control inflammation as effectively as possible, results in better outcomes than usual care. However, a DAS28 is not available at most visits, as a joint count is not usually performed.[52]

One approach to introduce clinical measurement into standard rheumatology care involves provision of incentives to a rheumatologist to collect quantitative measures, such as increasing reimbursement or as a direct requirement to prescribe a certain therapy for a particular patient. A second approach might involve using a simple patient self-report questionnaire at all visits, which involves no additional effort for the physicians and health professional, other than review. The questionnaire could be scored and reviewed in 5 to 10 seconds, and would be regarded as adding to, rather than interfering with, a standard clinical visit.

A multidimensional health assessment questionnaire (MDHAQ)[53,54] has been developed in usual patient care. Although reported primarily in RA, the MDHAQ has been useful clinically in patients with all rheumatic diseases.[55,56] A patient questionnaire may be regarded as a standardized, quantitative, scientific patient history (see "Patient Questionnaires in Rheumatoid Arthritis: Advantages and Limitations as a Quantitative, Standardized Scientific Medical History," by Pincus T, et al, in this issue). Information from a patient history is more important in management of most patients with rheumatic diseases than in most chronic diseases.

A compilation of scores on the modified health assessment questionnaire (MHAQ)— which anteceded the MDHAQ with only eight activities and a pain visual analog scale (VAS)[57]—was reported for patients seen by the corresponding author between 1982 and 1985. Scores were reported for five rheumatic diseases: 133 with RA, 206 with

Table 1
Mean levels of scores for physical function and pain at first visit in patients with any of five rheumatic diseases

	Number of Patients	Physical Function (0–10)[a]	Pain VAS (0–10)[b]	Physical Function: Rank	Pain Score: Rank
A. Patients seen 1982–1985[55]					
Rheumatoid arthritis (RA)	133	3.10	5.16	1	3
Osteoarthritis	206	1.87	6.01	3	2
Fibromyalgia	83	1.93	6.35	4	1
Systemic lupus erythematosus (SLE)	124	1.33	4.19	5	4
Systemic sclerosis	41	1.90	4.00	3	5
Adjusted P-value[c]	—	<0.001	<0.001	—	—
B. Patients seen 1996–2005[56]					
Rheumatoid arthritis (RA)	174	3.15	5.32	1	2
Osteoarthritis	32	1.75	4.30	4	3
Fibromyalgia	185	2.94	6.44	2	1
Systemic lupus erythematosus (SLE)	28	1.56	3.15	5	5
Systemic sclerosis	11	2.82	3.56	3	4

[a] Rheumatoid arthritis patients differ significantly (P<.01) from all other groups; systemic lupus erythematosus patients differ significantly (P<.01) from rheumatoid arthritis, osteoarthritis, and fibromyalgia patients.

[b] Osteoarthritis and fibromyalgia patients differ significantly (P<.05) from all other groups except one another.

[c] Overall statistical significance according to ANCOVA adjusted for age, duration of disease, race, sex, and formal education level.

Data from Callahan LF, Smith WJ, Pincus T. Self-report questionnaires in five rheumatic diseases: Comparisons of health status constructs and associations with formal education level. Arthritis Care Res 1989;2:122–31; Pincus T, Sokka T. Can a Multi-Dimensional Health Assessment Questionnaire (MDHAQ) and Routine Assessment of Patient Index Data (RAPID) scores be informative in patients with all rheumatic diseases? Best Pract Res Clin Rheumatol 2007;21:733–53.

Table 2
Summary of first recorded RAPID3 data collected in 867 patients at first visit seen 1996 to 2005 according to diagnosis

Diagnosis	N	Function		Pain		Global Estimate		Fatigue		RAPID3	
		Mean	Median	Mean	Median	Mean	Median	Mean	Median	Mean	Median
1-Rheumatoid arthritis	174	3.15	3.00	5.32	5.35	5.25	5.35	5.58	6.20	4.58	4.64
2-Inflammatory arthritis	151	2.02	1.67	4.88	4.90	4.43	4.30	5.01	4.80	3.78	3.52
3-Psoriatic arthritis	17	2.69	2.67	5.47	5.80	5.03	4.90	4.02	4.80	4.40	4.61
4-Systemic lupus erythematosus	28	1.56	1.17	3.15	2.55	3.90	4.70	5.07	5.45	2.87	2.85
5-Systemic sclerosis	11	2.82	2.00	3.56	3.60	4.97	4.90	4.76	6.00	3.78	3.50
6-Vasculitis	8	1.54	1.34	3.45	3.05	3.85	4.40	5.50	5.55	2.95	3.30
7-Osteoarthritis	32	1.75	1.67	4.30	5.15	3.97	4.45	3.39	3.10	3.34	3.48
8-Fibromyalgia	185	2.94	3.00	6.44	6.70	6.11	6.30	7.29	7.90	5.17	5.32
9-Other	261	1.95	1.33	4.52	4.60	4.35	4.40	4.47	4.50	3.61	3.40
Total	867	2.42	2.00	5.10	5.40	4.91	5.00	5.37	5.70	4.14	4.18

Data from Pincus T, Sokka T. Can a Multi-Dimensional Health Assessment Questionnaire (MDHAQ) and Routine Assessment of Patient Index Data (RAPID) scores be informative in patients with all rheumatic diseases? Best Pract Res Clin Rheumatol 2007;21:733–53.

osteoarthritis, 83 with fibromyalgia, 124 with SLE, and 41 with systemic sclerosis (**Table 1**).[55] Mean physical function scores on a 0 to10 scale (adjusted from a 1–4 scale used at that time) ranged from 1.33 in SLE to 3.10 in RA. Mean pain VAS scores on a 0 to10 scale ranged from 4.00 in systemic sclerosis to 6.35 in fibromyalgia (**Table 1A**). The table presents mean scores, and individual patients vary considerably. Nonetheless, the data indicate that scores for physical function and pain are elevated in most patients with all rheumatic diseases.

A similar compilation of all new patients seen by the corresponding author between 1996 and 2005, including 174 with RA, 32 with osteoarthritis, 185 with fibromyalgia, 28 with SLE, and 11 with systemic sclerosis, is presented in the lower panel of **Table 1B**.[56] Mean baseline scores for physical function ranged from 1.56 in SLE to 3.15 in RA, and indicated similar patterns to those in patients seen two decades earlier. Mean pain scores ranged from 3.15 in SLE to 6.44 in fibromyalgia, also similar to scores seen in the earlier cohort. Again, the data indicate the value of baseline MDHAQ scores in rheumatic diseases other than RA.

Further details concerning mean and median scores for physical function, pain, global estimate of status, fatigue, and routine assessment of patient index data (RAPID3)[20]—an index comprising of the first three measures (ie, the three patient-reported measures from the RA Core Data Set[58])—are illustrated in **Table 2** for 867 patients at their first visit between 1996 and 2005.[56] **Table 2** includes patients depicted in **Table 1B** as well as patients with inflammatory arthritis, psoriatic arthritis, and vasculitis. Overall, median scores for all patients were 2.00 for physical function, 5.40 for pain, 5.00 for global estimate, 5.70 for fatigue, and 4.18 for RAPID3, indicating that most patients with all rheumatologic diagnoses have abnormal scores. Highest scores were seen in patients with fibromyalgia for all three VAS components (pain, global estimate, fatigue) and for RAPID3. Lowest scores on all scales were seen in patients with vasculitis. A high score for pain with lower scores for physical function was seen in patients with osteoarthritis compared with RA, and inflammatory and psoriatic arthritis. Patients with SLE had higher global scores and lower pain scores than patients with osteoarthritis, although they were younger patients.

In osteoarthritis clinical trials, the physical function scale on the MDHAQ was more sensitive to changes than traditional physical nonquestionnaire measures.[59] A pain VAS on the MDHAQ is more sensitive than the Western Ontario McMaster osteoarthritis index (WOMAC)[60] to distinguish diclofenac and misoprostol from acetaminophen[61] or celecoxib from acetaminophen.[62] Furthermore, in fibromyalgia, ratios of pain or fatigue to physical function scores, and the number of symptoms reported on a checklist for review of systems, distinguish these patients from those with RA as effectively as ESR.[63,64]

The MDHAQ was adapted from the HAQ for feasibility in usual clinical care. Of course, it would be desirable to complete a complex index at every visit of a patient with SLE, systemic sclerosis, or other rheumatic disease, but this rarely occurs in usual care. Although less comprehensive or specific than a complex index, quantitative data on an MDHAQ appear preferable to no quantitative clinical data at all (other than laboratory tests).

Routine completion of an MDHAQ by every patient at every visit in the infrastructure of standard rheumatology care[65] allows quantitative monitoring of clinical status effectively, with minimal work on the part of the physician and the staff. The corresponding author has empirically collected MDHAQ scores to monitor clinical status in every patient (with any rheumatic disease) since 1982. Scores for physical function, pain, global estimate of status, and RAPID3—which have been termed "vital signs" for review in each patient at each visit to a rheumatologist—can function effectively for treatment of patients with all rheumatic diseases.

REFERENCES

1. Arnett FC, Edworthy SM, Bloch DA, et al. The American Rheumatism Association 1987 revised criteria for the classification of rheumatoid arthritis. Arthritis Rheum 1988;31:315–24.
2. Dougados M, van der Linden S, Juhlin R, et al. The European spondylarthropathy study group preliminary criteria for the classification of spondylarthropathy. Arthritis Rheum 1991;34:1218–27.
3. Special Writing Group of the Committee on Rheumatic Fever, Endocarditis, and Kawasaki Disease of the Council on Cardiovascular Disease in the Young, American Heart Association. Guidelines for the diagnosis of rheumatic fever: Jones criteria, updated 1992. JAMA 1992;268:2069–73.
4. Altman R, Alarcon G, Appelrouth D, et al. The American College of Rheumatology criteria for the classification and reporting of osteoarthritis of the hand. Arthritis Rheum 1990;33:1601–10.
5. Altman R, Alarcon G, Appelrouth D, et al. The American College of Rheumatology criteria for the classification of osteoarthritis of the hip. Arthritis Rheum 1991;34:505–14.
6. Wallace SL, Robinson H, Masi AT, et al. Preliminary criteria for the classification of the acute arthritis of primary gout. Arthritis Rheum 1977;20:895–900.
7. Tan EM, Cohen AS, Fries JF, et al. The 1982 revised criteria for the classification of systematic lupus erythematosus. Arthritis Rheum 1982;25:1271–7.
8. Hochberg MC. Updating the American College of Rheumatology revised criteria for the classification of systemic lupus erythematosus [letter]. Arthritis Rheum 1997;40:1725.
9. Masi AT, Rodnan GP, Medsger TA. Subcommittee for Scleroderma Criteria of the American Rheumatism Association Diagnostic and Therapeutic Criteria Committee. Preliminary criteria for the classification of systemic sclerosis (scleroderma). Arthritis Rheum 1980;23:581–90.
10. Bohan A, Peter JB. Polymyositis and dermatomyositis. N Engl J Med 1975;292:344–7, 403–7.
11. Vitali C, Bombardieri S, Moutsopoulos HM, et al. Preliminary criteria for the classification of Sjogren's syndrome. Results of a prospective concerted action supported by the European Community. Arthritis Rheum 1993;36:340–7.
12. Calabrese LH, Michel BA, Bloch DA, et al. The American College of Rheumatology 1990 criteria for the classification of hypersensitivity vasculitis. Arthritis Rheum 1990;33:1108–13.
13. International Study Group for Behçet's Disease. Criteria for diagnosis of Behçet's disease. Lancet 1990;335:1078–80.
14. Wilson WA, Gharavi AE, Koike T, et al. International consensus statement on preliminary classification criteria for definite antiphospholipid syndrome: report of an international workshop. Arthritis Rheum 1999;42:1309–11.
15. van der Heijde DM, van't Hof M, van Riel PL, et al. Development of a disease activity score based on judgment in clinical practice by rheumatologists. J Rheumatol 1993;20:579–81.
16. Prevoo ML, van't Hof MA, Kuper HH, et al. Modified disease activity scores that include twenty-eight-joint counts: development and validation in a prospective longitudinal study of patients with rheumatoid arthritis. Arthritis Rheum 1995;38:44–8.

17. Aletaha D, Smolen J. The simplified disease activity index (SDAI) and the clinical disease activity index (CDAI): a review of their usefulness and validity in rheumatoid arthritis. Clin Exp Rheumatol 2005;23:S100–8.
18. Pincus T, Strand V, Koch G, et al. An index of the three core data set patient questionnaire measures distinguishes efficacy of active treatment from placebo as effectively as the American College of Rheumatology 20% response criteria (ACR20) or the disease activity score (DAS) in a rheumatoid arthritis clinical trial. Arthritis Rheum 2003;48:625–30.
19. Pincus T, Bergman MJ, Yazici Y, et al. An index of only patient-reported outcome measures, routine assessment of patient index data 3 (RAPID3), in two abatacept clinical trials: similar results to disease activity score (DAS28) and other RAPID indices that include physician-reported measures. Rheumatology (Oxford) 2008;47:345–9.
20. Pincus T, Swearingen CJ, Bergman M, et al. RAPID3 (routine assessment of patient index data 3), a rheumatoid arthritis index without formal joint counts for routine care: proposed severity categories compared to DAS and CDAI categories. J Rheumatol 2008;35:2136–47.
21. Petri M, Hellmann DB, Hochberg M. Validity and reliability of lupus activity measures in the routine clinic setting. J Rheumatol 1992;19:53–9.
22. Bencivelli W, Vitali C, Isenberg DA, et al. Disease activity in systemic lupus erythematosus: report of the Consensus Study Group of the European Workshop for Rheumatology Research. III. Development of a computerised clinical chart and its application to the comparison of different indices of disease activity. The European Consensus Study Group for Disease Activity in SLE. Clin Exp Rheumatol 1992;10:549–54.
23. Hawker G, Gabriel S, Bombardier C, et al. A reliability study of SLEDAI: a disease activity index for systemic lupus erythematosus. J Rheumatol 1993;20:657–60.
24. Hay EM, Bacon PA, Gordon C, et al. The BILAG index: a reliable and valid instrument for measuring clinical disease activity in systemic lupus erythematosus. Q J Med 1993;86:447–58.
25. Gladman DD, Urowitz MB, Goldsmith CH, et al. The reliability of the Systemic Lupus International Collaborating Clinics/American College of Rheumatology damage index in patients with systemic lupus erythematosus. Arthritis Rheum 1997;40:809–13.
26. Mosca M, Bencivelli W, Vitali C, et al. The validity of the ECLAM index for the retrospective evaluation of disease activity in systemic lupus erythematosus. Lupus 2000;9:445–50.
27. Swaak AJ, van den Brink HG, Smeenk RJ, et al. Systemic lupus erythematosus. Disease outcome in patients with a disease duration of at least 10 years: second evaluation. Lupus 2001;10:51–8.
28. Lam GKW, Petri M. Assessment of systemic lupus erythematosus. Clin Exp Rheumatol 2005;23:S120–32.
29. Luqmani RA, Bacon PA, Moots RJ, et al. Birmingham Vasculitis Activity Score (BVAS) in systemic necrotizing vasculitis. Q J Med 1994;87:671–8.
30. Bacon PA, Moots RJ, Exley E, et al. VITAL assessment of vasculitis: workshop report. Clin Exp Rheumatol 1995;13:275–8.
31. Exley AR, Bacon PA, Luqmani RA, et al. Development and initial validation of the Vasculitis Damage Index for the standardized clinical assessment of damage in the systemic vasculitides. Arthritis Rheum 1997;40:371–80.
32. Whiting O'Keefe QE, Stone JH, Hellmann DB. Validity of a vasculitis activity index for systemic necrotizing vasculitis. Arthritis Rheum 1999;42:2365–71.

33. Stone JH, Hoffman GS, Merkel PA, et al. A disease-specific activity index for Wegener's granulomatosis: modification of the Birmingham Vasculitis Activity Score. Arthritis Rheum 2001;44:912–20.
34. Seo P, Min Y, Holbrook JT, et al. Damage caused by Wegener's granulomatosis and its treatment: prospective data from the Wegener's Granulomatosis Etanercept Trail (WGET). Arthritis Rheum 2005;52:2168–78.
35. Clegg DO, Reda DJ, Weisman MH, et al. Comparison of sulfasalazine and placebo in the treatment of ankylosing spondylitis. A Department of Veterans Affairs Cooperative Study. Arthritis Rheum 1996;39:2004–12.
36. Fleischer JAB, Feldman SR, Rapp SR, et al. Disease severity measures in a population of psoriasis patients: the symptoms of psoriasis correlate with self-administered psoriasis area severity index scores. J Invest Dermatol 1996;107:26–9.
37. Kavanaugh A, Cassell S. The assessment of disease activity and outcomes in psoriatic arthritis. Clin Exp Rheumatol 2005;23:S142–7.
38. Dougados M, Gueguen A, Nakache JP, et al. Evaluation of a functional index and an articular index in ankylosing spondylitis. J Rheumatol 1988;15:302–7.
39. Calin A, Garrett S, Whitelock H, et al. A new approach to defining functional ability in ankylosing spondylitis: the development of the Bath Ankylosing Spondylitis Functional Index. J Rheumatol 1994;21:2281–5.
40. Calin A, Nakache JP, Gueguen A, et al. Defining disease activity in ankylosing spondylitis: is a combination of variables (Bath Ankylosing Spondylitis Disease Activity Index) an appropriate instrument? Rheumatology (Oxford) 1999;38:878–82.
41. Calin A, MacKay K, Santos H, et al. A new dimension to outcome: application of the Bath Ankylosing Spondylitis Radiology Index. J Rheumatol 1999;26:988–92.
42. Zochling J, Braun J. Assessment of ankylosing spondylitis. Clin Exp Rheumatol 2005;23:S133–41.
43. Wolfe F, Michaud K. The clinical and research significance of the erythrocyte sedimentation rate. J Rheumatol 1994;21:1227–37.
44. Wolfe F, Pincus T. The level of inflammation in rheumatoid arthritis is determined early and remains stable over the longterm course of the illness. J Rheumatol 2001;28:1817–24.
45. Pincus T. Advantages and limitations of quantitative measures to assess rheumatoid arthritis: joint counts, radiographs, laboratory tests, and patient questionnaires. Bull Hosp Joint Dis 2006;64:32–9.
46. Möttönen T, Hannonen P, Leirisalo-Repo M, et al. Comparison of combination therapy with single-drug therapy in early rheumatoid arthritis: a randomised trial. FIN-RACo trial group. Lancet 1999;353:1568–73.
47. Grigor C, Capell H, Stirling A, et al. Effect of a treatment strategy of tight control for rheumatoid arthritis (the TICORA study): a single-blind randomised controlled trial. Lancet 2004;364:263–9.
48. Goekoop-Ruiterman YPM, de Vries-Bouwstra JK, Allaart CF, et al. Comparison of treatment strategies in early rheumatoid arthritis: a randomized trial. Ann Intern Med 2007;146:406–15.
49. Verstappen SMM, Jacobs JWG, van der Veen MJ, et al. Intensive treatment with methotrexate in early rheumatoid arthritis: aiming for remission. Computer Assisted Management in Early Rheumatoid Arthritis (CAMERA, an open-label strategy trial). Ann Rheum Dis 2007;66:1443–9.
50. Hetland ML, Stengaard-Pedersen K, Junker P, et al. Aggressive combination therapy with intra-articular glucocorticoid injections and conventional

disease-modifying anti-rheumatic drugs in early rheumatoid arthritis: second-year clinical and radiographic results from the CIMESTRA study. Ann Rheum Dis 2008;67:815–22.

51. Saunders SA, Capell HA, Stirling A, et al. Triple therapy in early active rheumatoid arthritis: a randomized, single-blind, controlled trial comparing step-up and parallel treatment strategies. Arthritis Rheum 2008;58:1310–7.

52. Pincus T, Segurado OG. Most visits of most patients with rheumatoid arthritis to most rheumatologists do not include a formal quantitative joint count. Ann Rheum Dis 2006;65:820–2.

53. Pincus T, Swearingen C, Wolfe F. Toward a multidimensional health assessment questionnaire (MDHAQ): assessment of advanced activities of daily living and psychological status in the patient friendly health assessment questionnaire format. Arthritis Rheum 1999;42:2220–30.

54. Pincus T, Sokka T, Kautiainen H. Further development of a physical function scale on a multidimensional health assessment questionnaire for standard care of patients with rheumatic diseases. J Rheumatol 2005;32:1432–9.

55. Callahan LF, Smith WJ, Pincus T. Self-report questionnaires in five rheumatic diseases: comparisons of health status constructs and associations with formal education level. Arthritis Care Res 1989;2:122–31.

56. Pincus T, Sokka T. Can a Multi-Dimensional Health Assessment Questionnaire (MDHAQ) and Routine Assessment of Patient Index Data (RAPID) scores be informative in patients with all rheumatic diseases? Best Pract Res Clin Rheumatol 2007;21:733–53.

57. Pincus T, Summey JA, Soraci SA Jr, et al. Assessment of patient satisfaction in activities of daily living using a modified Stanford health assessment questionnaire. Arthritis Rheum 1983;26:1346–53.

58. Felson DT, Anderson JJ, Boers M, et al. The American College of Rheumatology preliminary core set of disease activity measures for rheumatoid arthritis clinical trials. Arthritis Rheum 1993;36:729–40.

59. Brooks RH, Callahan LF, Pincus T. Use of self-report activities of daily living questionnaires in osteoarthritis. Arthritis Care Res 1988;1:23–32.

60. Bellamy N, Buchanan WW, Goldsmith CH, et al. Validation study of WOMAC: a health status instrument for measuring clinically important patient relevant outcomes to antirheumatic drug therapy in patients with osteoarthritis of the hip or knee. J Rheumatol 1988;15:1833–40.

61. Pincus T, Koch GG, Sokka T, et al. A randomized, double-blind, crossover clinical trial of diclofenac plus misoprostol versus acetaminophen in patients with osteoarthritis of the hip or knee. Arthritis Rheum 2001;44:1587–98.

62. Pincus T, Koch G, Lei H, et al. Patient preference for placebo, acetaminophen or celecoxib efficacy studies (PACES): two randomized placebo-controlled crossover clinical trials in patients with osteoarthritis of the knee or hip. Ann Rheum Dis 2004;63:931–9.

63. DeWalt DA, Reed GW, Pincus T. Further clues to recognition of patients with fibromyalgia from a simple 2-page patient multidimensional health assessment questionnaire (MDHAQ). Clin Exp Rheumatol 2004;22:453–61.

64. Callahan LF, Pincus T. The P-VAS/D-ADL ratio: a clue from a self-report questionnaire to distinguish rheumatoid arthritis from noninflammatory diffuse musculoskeletal pain. Arthritis Rheum 1990;33:1317–22.

65. Pincus T, Wolfe F. An infrastructure of patient questionnaires at each rheumatology visit: Improving efficiency and documenting care. J Rheumatol 2000;27:2727–30.

Flowsheets That Include MDHAQ Physical Function, Pain, Global, and RAPID3 Scores, Laboratory Tests, and Medications to Monitor Patients with all Rheumatic Diseases: An Electronic Database for an Electronic Medical Record

Theodore Pincus, MD[a],*, Arthur M. Mandelin II, MD, PhD[b],
Christopher J. Swearingen, PhD[c]

KEYWORDS

- Electronic medical record • Flowsheet
- Multidimensional health assessment questionnaire (MDHAQ)
- Routine assessment of patient index data (RAPID3)

An electronic medical record (EMR) has been introduced into many medical settings over the last decade. The EMR allows laboratory test results to be downloaded directly into a medical record to be available immediately at the site of patient care. The EMR may include direct entry of prescriptions, which can be submitted

A version of this article originally appeared in the 21:4 issue of *Best Practice & Research: Clinical Rheumatology*.

[a] Division of Rheumatology, NYU Hospital for Joint Diseases, 301 East 17th Street, Room 1608, New York, NY 10003, USA
[b] Division of Rheumatology, Department of Medicine, Feinberg School of Medicine, Northwestern University, Chicago, IL, USA
[c] Department of Pediatrics, Biostatistics Program, University of Arkansas for Medical Sciences, Little Rock, AR, USA
* Corresponding author.
E-mail address: tedpincus@gmail.com (T. Pincus).

electronically to a pharmacy, are difficult to lose, and are identical in the medical record and the pharmacy. The EMR is available at all times, from multiple locations, unlikely to be lost, and resolves problems of poor penmanship.

An EMR requires a computer, suggesting to some observers that information in the EMR is available for analyses of patient care, results of different types of treatments, and long-term outcomes. Laboratory and medication data in an EMR may be in an electronic database, but most components of an EMR are narratives, analogous to Microsoft Word, rather than Excel or Access files. Although entry into a computer is performed, the information in the narrative is not segregated into machine-readable discrete data points to be available for analyses.

It is no more difficult to enter the same data into a database for analyses as into a narrative word-processing program. The structure of a database, however, must be established in advance. Because information from patients is particularly prominent in clinical decisions by rheumatologists, a database structure for monitoring patients with rheumatic diseases should include data from a patient history, collected as standardized, quantitative scientific data on a patient self-report questionnaire. At this time, most available EMRs do not include the capacity to enter patient questionnaire data, and cannot be used to determine quantitatively whether patients with rheumatic diseases are better, worse, or the same from one visit to another, or over longer periods.

The corresponding author has implemented a database on all patient visits since 1980, converted to Microsoft Access software in 2000, which includes patient questionnaire, laboratory, and medication data from each visit. A multidimensional health assessment questionnaire (MDHAQ)[1,2] is completed by each patient at each visit, allowing recording of scores for physical function; pain; global estimate of status; and Routine Assessment of Patient Index Data (RAPID3),[3,4] a composite index of the three individual measures. RAPID3 is scored 0 to 30; scores may be classified as indicating high (>12), moderate (6.1–12), and low (3.1–6) severity, and near remission (≤3).[3,4] These data can be entered into an electronic flowsheet to be monitored along with laboratory test results and medications.

Flowsheets have been generated for each patient visit since 2000. The MDHAQ, laboratory, and medication data are entered by a secretary; an automated letter is generated by the database. **Figs. 1** to **11** illustrate clinical courses over periods varying from a few months to 15 years in patients with different diagnoses other than rheumatoid arthritis, to illustrate the value of monitoring scores for the three Core Data Set MDHAQ measures and RAPID3 over time in all patients seen in standard rheumatology clinical care. Visit dates have been randomly altered slightly to preserve privacy, but reflect the actual time course of the patient histories; months and years are unchanged.

DISCUSSION

The flowsheets presented in this article of 11 patients who did not have rheumatoid arthritis were selected to illustrate that the MDHAQ and RAPID3 can be informative in patients with all rheumatic diseases. Thus, data from the same patient questionnaire can be helpful in formulating clinical decisions and documenting results of care in patients with any rheumatic disease. The flowsheets illustrate that patient questionnaire scores may be regarded as quantitative data, analogous to laboratory tests or vital signs (see article by Pincus T, Yazici Y, Bergman MB, in this issue). If the clinician has available questionnaire scores before seeing the patient, particularly comparative data from previous visits on a flowsheet, evidence of a RAPID3 score (0–30 scale) in

Multi-Dimensional Health Assessment Questionnaire (MDHAQ) Scores, Laboratory Tests, Medications
DOB: _April 1980_ 1st Visit: _26 May 2004_ DX ICD9: _696.00_ Onset: _Oct 2003_ Education: _16_

VISIT DATE	26 May 04	4 Jun 04	9 Sept 04	16 Dec 04	15 Apr 05	24 Oct 05	26 Jun 06
PATIENT SELF-REPORT QUESTIONNAIRE DATA							
FUNCTIONAL STATUS (FN) [0-10]	4.0	2.0	1.0	2.0	0.7	0	0.3
PAIN (PN) [0-10]	7.6	2.5	2.5	4.1	1.1	0	0.8
GLOBAL STATUS (GL) [0-10]	6.5	2.1	1.6	6.9	2.8	1	0.8
RAPID3 (0-30)	18.1	6.6	5.1	13.0	3.9	1	1.9
PHYSICAL MEASURES DATA							
WEIGHT (lbs)	NA	136	136	135	136	137	142
BLOOD PRESSURE (mm/Hg)	NA	128/72	117/70	131/78	114/66	113/69	131/85
LABORATORY DATA							
ESR (mm/hr) [M:0-20 / F:0-30]		12	4			9	3
CRP (mg/L) [0-10]		6	3	3.2		1.5	0.9
WBC (thou/uL) [4-11]	10.7	6.7	13.2	12.3		7.5	7.0
HGB (g/dL) [M:14-18/F:12-16]	12.4	14.5	14.9	15.5		15.4	14.7
HCT (%) [M:42-50/F:37-44]	37	40	45	45		43	42
PLATELETS (thou/uL) [150-400]	436	268	383	401		335	363
ALBUMIN (g/dL) [3.5-5.0]		4.7	4.5		4.5	4.9	5.1
ALK PHOS (U/L) [40-100]		75		62	86		68
SGOT (U/L) [4-40]		78	72		64	59	79
CREATININE (mg/dL) [0.7-1.5]		18	17		29	24	26
RHEUMATOLOGY MEDICATIONS (C=Change Dose, D=D/C, N=New, O=On at visit, P=Parenteral, R=Resume, S=Short Term, T=Taper)							
Prednisone	O-20 QD	T-19 QD	T-9 QD	W-6 QD	W-3 QD	D	N-3 QD
Methotrexate	O-10 QW	O-10 QW	C-10 QW	C-5 QW	W-5 QW	W-5 QW	W-5 QW
Folic Acid	O-1 QD	O-1 QD	W-1 QD	W-1 QD	W-1 QD	W-1 QD	W-1 QD
Rofecoxib	O-50 QD	C-25 QD	D				
Adalimumab				N-40 Q2W	W-40 Q2W	W-40 Q2W	W-40 Q2W

Fig. 1. Psoriatic arthritis in a 24-year-old woman. A 24-year-old female patient was seen in an emergency room for a swollen right elbow on May 26, 2004. An arthrocentesis revealed milky fluid and the patient was admitted for presumed septic arthritis. She did not improve with antibiotic therapy on the second day, and a rheumatologist was called. The rheumatologist elicited a history of mild psoriasis and polyarthralgias over the previous 2 years, and made a diagnosis of psoriatic arthritis. The patient's MDHAQ scores were 4 (0–10) for physical function, pain 7.6 (0–10), global status 6.5 (0–10), and RAPID3 was 18.1 on a 0–30 scale, indicating high severity (RAPID3>12). She was treated with 20 mg prednisone daily and 10 mg methotrexate per week. By June 4, 2004, her functional status had improved to 2, pain to 2.5, global status to 2.1, and RAPID3 (0–30 scale) to 6.6, indicating moderate severity (6.1–12). On September 9, 2004, RAPID3 was 5.1, indicating mild severity (3.1–6). On December 16, 2004, she experienced a flare; her score for physical function rose to 2, pain to 4.1, global status to 6.9, and RAPID3 to 13, indicating high severity again. After discussion with the patient and her family, it was elected to begin adalimumab, 40 mg, every other week. Ten months later, on October 24, 2005, her functional status score was 0, pain 0, global status 1, and RAPID3 1, indicating near remission (≤3). Her scores remained stable over the following year. (*Courtesy of* Health Report Services. Copyright © 2009 Health Reports Service, Inc. Email: tedpincus@gmail.com.)

Multi-Dimensional Health Assessment Questionnaire (MDHAQ) Scores, Laboratory Tests, Medications
DOB: _Aug 1965_ 1st Visit: _14 Feb 2005_ DX ICD9: _710.10_ Onset: _Sept 2004_ Education: _12_

VISIT DATE	14 Feb 05	16 May 05	21 Jul 05	19 Sep 05	24 May 06	28 Sep 06	
PATIENT SELF-REPORT QUESTIONNAIRE DATA							
FUNCTIONAL STATUS (FN) [0-10]	4.3	0	0	0	0	0	
PAIN (PN) [0-10]	5.6	2	4	3.5	0.4	0.5	
GLOBAL STATUS (GL) [0-10]	6.5	6	3	2	0.1	0.5	
RAPID3 (0-30)	16.4	8	7	5.5	0.5	1	
PHYSICAL MEASURES DATA							
WEIGHT (lbs)	106	120	101	103	104	104	
BLOOD PRESSURE (mm/Hg)	132/74	170/94	153/75	143/84	116/60	115/70	
LABORATORY DATA							
ESR (mm/hr) [M:0-20 / F:0-30]	66	36		8	11	15	
CRP (mg/L) [0-10]	44.7		1.8	1.2	1	0.9	
WBC (thou/uL) [4-11]	4.3	8	6.8	5.1	5.6	4.1	
HGB (g/dL) [M:14-18/F:12-16]	10.8	10.6	12.6	13.8	12.9	13.1	
HCT (%) [M:42-50/F:37-44]	33	31	40	41	41	41	
PLATELETS (thou/uL) [150-400]	390	213	390	265	300	315	
ALBUMIN (g/dL) [3.5-5.0]	3.7	1.9		4.8	4.8	4.7	
ALK PHOS (U/L) [40-100]	108			74	86	91	
SGOT (U/L) [4-40]	21			17	15	19	
CREATININE (mg/dL) [0.7-1.5]	0.6	0.7	0.7	0.6	0.7	0.8	
RHEUMATOLOGY MEDICATIONS (C=Change Dose, D=D/C, N=New, O=On at visit, P=Parenteral, R=Resume, S=Short Term, T=Taper)							
Ibuprofen	O-600 TID	600 TID					
Prednisone	N-5 QD	C-10 QD	T-5QD	5 QD	C 4 QD	4 QD	
Methylprednisolone acetate	N-80						
Mycophenolate mofetil		N-500 BID	1000 BID	1000 BID	1000 BID	1000 BID	
Hydroxychloroquine				N-200 BID	D		

Fig. 2. Systemic lupus erythematosus in a 39-year-old woman. A 39-year-old woman was seen for pleuritis, pleural effusions, arthralgias, and positive tests for antinuclear antibody and anti-dsDNA antibodies on February 14, 2005. A diagnosis of systemic lupus erythematosus was made. Her score for physical function was 4.3, pain 5.6, global status 6.5, and RAPID3 16.4, indicating high severity (>12). She was treated with a prednisolone acetate injection, 80 mg, and oral prednisone, 5 mg per day, was begun. At her next visit of May 16, 2005, her score for functional status was 0, pain 2, global status 6, and RAPID3 8, indicating moderate severity (6.1–12), with improvement. She was given a prescription for mycophenolate mofetil, 500 mg twice a day. On July 21, 2005, her scores were 0 for physical function, 4 for pain, 3 for global status, and 7 for RAPID3, indicating moderate severity. Her mycophenolate mofetil was increased to 1000 mg twice a day and her prednisone was reduced to 5 mg every day. Over the next year, she showed considerable improvement, with scores on September 26, 2006, of 0 for physical function, 0.5 for pain, 0.5 for global status, and 1 for RAPID3, indicating near remission status (≤3). (*Courtesy of* Health Report Services. Copyright © 2009 Health Reports Service, Inc. Email: tedpincus@gmail.com.)

Multi-Dimensional Health Assessment Questionnaire (MDHAQ) Scores, Laboratory Tests, Medications
DOB: _Jan 1968_ 1ˢᵗ Visit: _11 Aug 2003_ DX ICD9: _720.00_ Onset: _Jan 1990_ Education: _10_

VISIT DATE	11 Aug 03	27 Aug 03	24 Sep 03	24 Nov 03	18 Mar 04	14 Mar 05	7 Sep 06
PATIENT SELF-REPORT QUESTIONNAIRE DATA							
FUNCTIONAL STATUS **(FN)** [0-10]	5.7	4.7	6.3	3.7	3.3	3.7	3.3
PAIN **(PN)** [0-10]	8.8	5.2	8.8	0.6	0.2	0.2	0.5
GLOBAL STATUS **(GL)** [0-10]	4.9	3.5	5.0	2.4	0.3	0.3	0.5
RAPID3 (0-30)	19.4	13.4	20.1	6.7	3.8	4.2	4.3
PHYSICAL MEASURES DATA							
WEIGHT (lbs)	158	160	162.6	181	180	189	220
BLOOD PRESSURE (mm/Hg)	122/80	126/76	129/78	133/80	130.78	139/76	130/82
LABORATORY DATA							
ESR (mm/hr) [M:0-20 / F:0-30]	17		39	8	4	6	13
CRP (mg/L) [0-10]	36		67	2	7	3.4	20.3
WBC (thou/uL) [4-11]	14.5		11.2	9.7	9.8	9.3	8.6
HGB (g/dL) [M:14-18/F:12-16]	15		14.3	14.4	15.6	16.6	14.1
HCT (%) [M:42-50/F:37-44]	45		45	44	48	48	44
PLATELETS (thou/uL) [150-400]	373		338	213	218	235	227
ALBUMIN (g/dL) [3.5-5.0]	4.4		4.5		4.4	4.5	4.3
ALK PHOS (U/L) [40-100]	94		93		73	69	87
SGOT (U/L) [4-40]	17		17		29	20	21
CREATININE (mg/dL) [0.7-1.5]	0.7			0.7	0.7	0.8	0.7
RHEUMATOLOGY MEDICATIONS (C=Change Dose, D=D/C, N=New, O=On at visit, P=Parenteral, R=Resume, S=Short Term, T=Taper)							
Prednisone	N-5 QD	5 QD	5 QD	T-4 QD	4 QD	4 QD	D-4 QD
Phenylbutazone	N-300 QD	300 QD	300 QD	300 QD	D-300QD		
Methotrexate		N-10 QW	C-20 QW	20 QW	D-20QW	10 QW	D
Folic Acid		N-1 QD	1 QD	1 QD	D-1 QD	1 QD	D
Etanercept			N-25 BIW	25 BIW	25 BIW	25 BIW	25 BIW

Fig. 3. Ankylosing spondylitis in a 35-year-old man. A 35-year-old man was seen on August 11, 2003, for severe back pain, seeking disability status from his work as a carpenter. He related a history of back pain since age 24; however, a diagnosis of ankylosing spondylitis had been made only 2 weeks earlier by his family physician. Physical examination revealed a marked kyphosis and flexion contractures of both hips and both knees, with obvious ankylosing spondylitis. His scores were 5.7 for physical function, 8.8 for pain, 4.9 for global status, and 19.4 for RAPID3, indicating high severity (>12). He was treated with prednisone, 5 mg per day, and phenylbutazone, 300 mg per day. Two weeks later he had some improvement, with scores of 4.7 for physical function, 5.2 for pain, 3.5 for global status, and 13.4 for RAPID3, indicating persistent high severity. Methotrexate, 10 mg per week, was added. On September 24, 2003, however, the patient was clinically unchanged from his first visit, with recurrent high scores for functional status, pain, global status, and RAPID3 of 20.1, indicating persistent high severity. Etanercept, 25 mg twice weekly, was initiated. Two months later, on November 24, 2003, his score for physical function had improved from 6.3 to 3.7, pain from 8.8 to 0.6, global status from 5 to 2.4, and RAPID3 from 20.1 to 6.7, indicating moderate severity (6.1–12). Over the next 3 years, he maintained scores of less than 1 for pain and global status, although his physical function remained 3.3, and RAPID scores in the range of 3.8–4.3, indicating low severity (3.1–6), on the basis of damage from chronic ankylosing spondylitis over more than a decade before optimal treatment for his condition. He has continued to work as a carpenter, and participates in active weekend recreation, which he had given up before his treatment. (*Courtesy of* Health Report Services. Copyright © 2009 Health Reports Service, Inc. Email: tedpincus@gmail.com.)

Multi-Dimensional Health Assessment Questionnaire (MDHAQ) Scores, Laboratory Tests, Medications
DOB: _May 1935_ 1st Visit: _11 Dec 2003_ DX ICD9: _274.90_ Onset: _Jan 1973_ Education: _16_

VISIT DATE	11 Dec 03		9 Feb 04	18 Aug 04					
PATIENT SELF-REPORT QUESTIONNAIRE DATA									
FUNCTIONAL STATUS (FN) [0-10]	0.7		0	0					
PAIN (PN) [0-10]	4.3		0	0.5					
GLOBAL STATUS (GL) [0-10]	1.2		0	0.3					
RAPID3 (0-30)	6.2		0	0.8					
PHYSICAL MEASURES DATA									
WEIGHT (lbs)	198		201	194					
BLOOD PRESSURE (mm/Hg)	177/98		112/78	127/64					
LABORATORY DATA									
ESR (mm/hr) [M:0-20 / F:0-30]	5			3					
CRP (mg/L) [0-10]									
WBC (thou/uL) [4-11]	5.3		6.7	4.7					
HGB (g/dL) [M:14-18/F:12-16]	14.4		15	15.8					
HCT (%) [M:42-50/F:37-44]	42		44	45					
PLATELETS (thou/uL) [150-400]	178		208	186					
ALBUMIN (g/dL) [3.5-5.0]				4.7					
ALK PHOS (U/L) [40-100]				67					
SGOT (U/L) [4-40]				25					
CREATININE (mg/dL) [0.7-1.5]	1.1		1.1	1.1					
RHEUMATOLOGY MEDICATIONS (C=Change Dose, D=D/C, N=New, O=On at visit, P=Parenteral, R=Resume, S=Short Term, T=Taper)									
Prednisone	N-5 QD		D-5QD						
Allopurinol	N-300 QD		300 QD	300 QD					
Colchicine	R-0.6 QD		0.6 QD	D					
Propanolol hydrochloride	O-10 QD		10 QD	10 QD					

Fig. 4. Gout in a 68-year-old man. A 68-year-old man was seen because of chronic gout with a recent acute attack on December 11, 2003, referred from the emergency department. His attack had abated, although he had some residual erythema of his right great toe. His MDHAQ scores were 0.7 for physical function, 4.3 for pain, 1.2 for global status, and 6.2 for RAPID3, indicating moderate severity (6.1–12). He was treated with prednisone, 5 mg per day, allopurinol, 300 mg per day, and colchicine, 0.6 mg per day. Two months later, on February 9, 2004, his scores were all 0, indicating near remission (≤3). His prednisone was discontinued, and allopurinol and colchicine were continued. On August 18, 2004, his score for physical function was 0, pain 0.5, global status 0.3, and RAPID3 0.8, indicating continued near remission status. His colchicine was discontinued and he was returned to the care of his family physician. (*Courtesy of* Health Report Services. Copyright © 2009 Health Reports Service, Inc. Email: tedpincus@gmail.com.)

Multi-Dimensional Health Assessment Questionnaire (MDHAQ) Scores, Laboratory Tests, Medications
DOB: _Mar 1947_ 1st Visit: _9 Sep 1992_ DX ICD9: _710.10_ Onset: _July 1980_ Education: _16_

VISIT DATE	9 Sep 92	12 Nov 92	14 Jan 93	28 Oct 96	30 Jan 97	10 Jul 00	14 Sep 06
PATIENT SELF-REPORT QUESTIONNAIRE DATA							
FUNCTIONAL STATUS (FN) [0-10]	2.9	2.5	1.7	3.0	2.7	3.7	2.0
PAIN (PN) [0-10]	3.2	5.7	1	3	1.3	0.6	0.5
GLOBAL STATUS (GL) [0-10]				0.9	1.8	0.7	0
RAPID3 (0-30)	9.2*	12.3*	4.2*	6.9	5.8	5.0	2.5
PHYSICAL MEASURES DATA							
WEIGHT (lbs)	137	135	135	132	133	128	137
BLOOD PRESSURE (mm/Hg)	102/68	90/52	110/68	106/70	92/60	94/55	117/72
LABORATORY DATA							
ESR (mm/hr) [M:0-20 / F:0-30]	14		10	25	36	22	14
CRP (mg/L) [0-10]				1	3	5	0.6
WBC (thou/uL) [4-11]			5.2	6.3	7.4	6.1	6
HGB (g/dL) [M:14-18/F:12-16]							14
HCT (%) [M:42-50/F:37-44]			41	40	42	39	43
PLATELETS (thou/uL) [150-400]			106	151	212	168	145
ALBUMIN (g/dL) [3.5-5.0]			4	3.5	3.6	3.3	4.4
ALK PHOS (U/L) [40-100]			47	46	54	91	77
SGOT (U/L) [4-40]			13	18	20	28	30
CREATININE (mg/dL) [0.7-1.5]			0.8	0.7	0.9	0.9	0.9
RHEUMATOLOGY MEDICATIONS (C=Change Dose, D=D/C, N=New, O=On at visit, P=Parenteral, R=Resume, S=Short Term, T=Taper)							
Penicillamine	O-250 QD	250 QD	250 QD	625 QD	C-750 QD	750 QD	750 QD
Sulindac	O-200 QD	200 BID	200 BID	200 BID	200 BID	200 BID	200 BID
Prednisone		N-3 QD	3 QD	3 QD	3 QD	3 QD	3 QD
Methotrexate				7.5 QW	7.5 QW	C-5 QW	15 QW
Folic acid				1 QD	1 QD	1 QD	1 QD

*Estimated from sum of two scores (functional status and pain) multiplied by 1.5

Fig. 5. Systemic sclerosis in a 45-year-old woman. A 45-year-old woman with long-standing systemic sclerosis since age 33 was seen initially on September 9, 1992. Physical examination revealed classical proximal scleroderma with contractures of the PIP joints of both hands. Her score for physical function was 2.9, and pain was 3.2 (patient global scores were not obtained until 1995), indicating a RAPID3 score (intercalated) of 9.2, denoting moderate severity (6.1–12). She was treated with penicillamine, but showed no improvement on November 12, 1992, with worsening of her pain score to 5.7 and estimated RAPID3 score of 12.3, indicating high severity (>12). Prednisone, 3 mg per day, was added, resulting in a substantial improvement by January 14, 1993, with a pain score of 1 and RAPID3 score of 4.2, indicating low severity (3.1–6). She was stable until 1996, but experienced a flare on October 28, 1996, with a score for physical function of 3, pain of 3, global status of 0.9, and RAPID3 of 6.9, indicating moderate severity. Methotrexate, 10 mg per week, was added. She was maintained on low-dose prednisone, low-dose methotrexate, and penicillamine over many years, with maintenance of functional status and low pain scores. Her scores on September 14, 2006, were 2 for physical function, 0.5 for pain, 0 for global status, with RAPID3 of 2.5, indicating near-remission status (≤3). (*Courtesy of* Health Report Services. Copyright © 2009 Health Reports Service, Inc. Email: tedpincus@gmail.com.)

Multi-Dimensional Health Assessment Questionnaire (MDHAQ) Scores, Laboratory Tests, Medications
DOB: _July 1956_ 1st Visit: _15 Jan 1990_ DX ICD9: _447.60_ Onset: _July 1989_ Education: _12_

VISIT DATE	15 Jan 90	21 Mar 90	14 Aug 03	20 Dec 04	30 May 05	28 Nov 05	5 Jul 06	20 Sep 06
PATIENT SELF-REPORT QUESTIONNAIRE DATA								
FUNCTIONAL STATUS (FN) [0-10]	1.3	0.8	1.0	1.3	1.0	2.3	1.7	1.7
PAIN (PN) [0-10]	5.3	0.9	0.8	5.1	5	3	2.2	1.5
GLOBAL STATUS (GL) [0-10]	—	—	1.8	4.9	3	3.5	2.7	2.5
RAPID3 [0-30]	9.9*	2.5*	3.6	11.3	9	8.8	6.6	5.7
PHYSICAL MEASURES DATA								
WEIGHT (lbs)	113	117	124	131	132	153	159	156
BLOOD PRESSURE (mm/Hg)	110/70	120/90	97/65	127/71	111/77	143/90	131/86	120/79
LABORATORY DATA								
ESR (mm/hr) [M:0-20 / F:0-30]			12	17	38	16	9	13
CRP (mg/L) [0-10]			3		24.3	3.8	4.5	7.9
WBC (thou/uL) [4-11]		9.9	7.5	4.7		6.3	7.3	7.8
HGB (g/dL) [M:14-18/F:12-16]			15	13.4		13.9	14.5	14.2
HCT (%) [M:42-50/F:37-44]		34.5	44	38		43	44	44
PLATELETS (thou/uL) [150-400]		281	242	190		194	215	237
ALBUMIN (g/dL) [3.5-5.0]				3.8		4.2	4.3	4.6
GLUCOSE (mg/dL) [70-110]			93	123		111	206	169
ALK PHOS (U/L) [40-100]				70		72	92	103
SGOT (U/L) [4-40]				15		14	16	23
CREATININE (mg/dL) [0.7-1.5]			0.6	0.5		0.6	0.7	0.8
RHEUMATOLOGY MEDICATIONS (C=Change Dose, D=D/C, N=New, O=On at visit, P=Parenteral, R=Resume, S=Short Term, T=Taper)								
Cyclophosphamide	O-200 QD	R-50 QD			R-50 QD	C-100 QW	D	
Prednisone	O-30 QD	T-35 QD	2 QD	R-3 QD	3 QD	T-5 QD	5 QD	
Methotrexate			15 QW	R-10 QW	15 QW		R-15 QW	
Folic acid			1 QD	1 QD	1 QD	1 QD	1 QD	

*Estimated from sum of two scores (functional status and pain) multiplied by 1.5

Fig. 6. Vasculitis in a 34-year-old woman. A 34-year-old woman was seen on January 15, 1990, with palpable purpura, right foot drop, and hematuria. A diagnosis of vasculitis was made. Her score for functional disability was 1.3, pain was 5.3 (global scores were not obtained until 1995), and estimated RAPID3 score was 9.9, indicating moderate severity (6.1–12). She was treated with prednisone and cyclophosphamide over 1 year, then with methotrexate with substantial clinical improvement, and she was largely asymptomatic for 12 years, from 1991 to 2003. On August 14, 2003, her score for physical function was 1, pain 0.8, global status 1.8, and RAPID3 3.6, indicating low severity (3.1–6). She decided on her own to discontinue methotrexate in the fall of 2003. On December 20, 2004, she noted recurrent right foot drop and a new left foot drop. She had an increase in her score for physical function to 1.3, pain to 5.1, global status to 4.9, and RAPID3 to 11.3, indicating moderate severity (6.1–12). She was hospitalized and treated for 3 days with daily "pulse" methylprednisolone, 1000 mg per day, and showed gradual improvement. On May 30, 2005, however, she had a further exacerbation and was hospitalized and treated again with cyclophosphamide, which was maintained over 6 months. On November 28, 2005, her scores were 2.3 for physical function, 3 for pain, 3.5 for global status, and 8.8 for RAPID3, indicating persistent moderate severity (6.1–12). On July 5, 2006, RAPID3 was 6.6. Cyclophosphamide was discontinued, and methotrexate, 15 mg per week, was reinstated. On September 20, 2006, her score for physical function was 1.7, pain 1.5, global status 2.5, and RAPID3 5.7, indicating low severity (3.1–6). She was much improved, but had not recovered to her 1990–2003 level, as evidenced by RAPID3 of 5.7 compared with 3.6 in 2003. (*Courtesy of* Health Report Services. Copyright © 2009 Health Reports Service, Inc. Email: tedpincus@gmail.com.)

Multi-Dimensional Health Assessment Questionnaire (MDHAQ) Scores, Laboratory Tests, Medications
DOB: _Dec 1945_ 1ˢᵗ Visit: _29 Mar 1995_ DX ICD9: _729.10_ Onset: _July 1992_ Education: _12_

VISIT DATE	29 Mar 95	26 Jun 95	20 Dec 95				
PATIENT SELF-REPORT QUESTIONNAIRE DATA							
FUNCTIONAL STATUS (FN) [0-10]	2.67	0	0				
PAIN (PN) [0-10]	4.9	2.1	1.9				
GLOBAL STATUS (GL) [0-10]	–	–	–				
RAPID3 (0-30)	11.4*	3.2*	2.9*				
PHYSICAL MEASURES DATA							
WEIGHT (lbs)	206	180	148				
BLOOD PRESSURE (mm/Hg)	174/100	146/94	170/100				
LABORATORY DATA							
ESR (mm/hr) [M:0-20 / F:0-30]	15						
CRP (mg/L) [0-10]							
WBC (thou/uL) [4-11]	7.9						
HGB (g/dL) [M:14-18/F:12-16]	13.4						
HCT (%) [M:42-50/F:37-44]	38.8						
PLATELETS (thou/uL) [150-400]	285						
ALBUMIN (g/dL) [3.5-5.0]	4.5						
ALK PHOS (U/L) [40-100]	65						
SGOT (U/L) [4-40]	21						
CREATININE (mg/dL) [0.7-1.5]	0.8						
RHEUMATOLOGY MEDICATIONS (C=Change Dose, D=D/C, N=New, O=On at visit, P=Parenteral, R=Resume, S=Short Term, T=Taper)							
Nabumetone	O-750 BID	D					

*Estimated from sum of two scores (functional status and pain) multiplied by 1.5. (Patient global estimate of status not collected prior to 1996.)

Fig. 7. Fibromyalgia in a 49-year-old woman. A 49-year-old woman was seen on March 29, 1995, because of widespread musculoskeletal pain. She was a hairdresser who opened her beauty shop at 6 AM, although by temperament a "night person." Her scores were 2.7 for functional disability, 4.9 for pain, and estimated RAPID3 of 11.4, indicating moderate severity (6.1–12). She was advised to try to arrange for an employee to open her beauty shop in the morning, so that she could sleep until she naturally would awake at 8 AM, and to exercise by walking an hour per day. No new medications were prescribed. She was seen again 3 months later on June 26, 1995, with a weight loss of 26 pounds, improvement of her physical function score to 0 and pain to 2.1, and estimated RAPID3 score of 3.2, indicating low severity (3.1–6). She was seen again 6 months later on December 20, 1995, with a further loss of 32 pounds for a total of 58 pounds over 8 months. Her score for physical function was 0, pain 1.9, and estimated RAPID3 2.9, indicating near remission (≤3). This patient showed a very atypical response for patients with fibromyalgia, most of whom do not heed advice to exercise regularly (and do not show weight loss). The flowsheet documents her positive response. (*Courtesy of* Health Report Services. Copyright © 2009 Health Reports Service, Inc. Email: tedpincus@gmail.com.)

Multi-Dimensional Health Assessment Questionnaire (MDHAQ) Scores, Laboratory Tests, Medications
DOB: _July 1942_ 1st Visit: _27 May 1996_ DX ICD9: _729.10_ Onset: _July 1986_ Education: _12_

VISIT DATE	27 May 96	8 Jun 98	16 Jun 00	12 Dec 02	31 Jul 03	20 Oct 03	
PATIENT SELF-REPORT QUESTIONNAIRE DATA							
FUNCTIONAL STATUS (FN) [0-10]	0.7	2.3	2.7	3.0	5.0	0	
PAIN (PN) [0-10]	9.8	6.9	9.9	9.7	9.9	0.3	
GLOBAL STATUS (GL) [0-10]	—	5.8	9.5	8.6	9.6	0.1	
RAPID 3 (0-30)	15.8*	15.0	22.1	21.3	23.5	0.4	
PHYSICAL MEASURES DATA							
WEIGHT (lbs)	121	122	122	139	125	122	
BLOOD PRESSURE (mm/Hg)	140/90	138/70	152/76	174/84	172/89	160/80	
LABORATORY DATA							
ESR (mm/hr) [M:0-20 / F:0-30]	48				67		
CRP (mg/L) [0-10]	3						
WBC (thou/uL) [4-11]					6.6		
HGB (g/dL) [M:14-18/F:12-16]					11.1		
HCT (%) [M:42-50/F:37-44]					35		
PLATELETS (thou/uL) [150-400]					220		
ALBUMIN (g/dL) [3.5-5.0]	3.9				4		
ALK PHOS (U/L) [40-100]	85				106		
SGOT (U/L) [4-40]	18				32		
CREATININE (mg/dL) [0.7-1.5]	0.8				0.8		
RHEUMATOLOGY MEDICATIONS (C=Change Dose, D=D/C, N=New, O=On at visit, P=Parenteral, R=Resume, S=Short Term, T=Taper)							
Prednisone		3 QD	D-1 QD	5 QD	5 QD	D-5QD	
Celecoxib			100 BID				
Methotrexate				N-10 QW			
Depo-Medrol				40	40		
Valdecoxib						O-20 BID	
NON-RHEUMATOLOGY DRUGS (C=Change Dose, D=D/C, N=New, O=On at visit, R=Resume, S=Short Term, X=Tox							
Hydrocodone/APAP 5/500 tablet		4 QD	4 QD	C (next line)			
Hydrocodone/APAP 7.5/500 tablet				C-4 QD	4 QD	D	
Tramadol HCl	O-50 PRN						
Chloral hydrate		2 QD	2 QD	2 QD	2 QD	D	
Tramadol HCl	O-50 PRN						
Propoxyphene napsylate/APAP 100/650				O-1 PRN	1 PRN	D	
Triazolam		0.125 QD	D				
Amitriptyline		25 QHS	25 QHS	25 QHS	25 QHS	D	
Sertraline HCl						O-50 QD	
Zolpidem		15 QHS	15 QHS	15 QHS	20 QHS	D	

*Estimated from sum of two scores (functional status and pain) multiplied by 1.5
APAP = acetaminophen

Fig. 8. Fibromyalgia in a 53-year-old woman. A 53-year-old woman was seen initially on May 27, 1996, with a score for functional disability of 0.7, pain of 9.8, and estimated RAPID3 of 15.8, indicating high severity (>12). This pattern is typical of fibromyalgia, reflecting a high ratio of pain to functional status, which is virtually pathognomonic for fibromyalgia.[5,6] This patient had an erythrocyte sedimentation rate of 48 mm/h, and received an "n of 1" trial of low-dose prednisone, 3 to 5 mg over the years, which she said was helpful. She showed essentially no improvement in scores, however, and continued to take medications prescribed by other practitioners for pain, sleep, and mood disorders that included hydrocodone-acetaminophen, chloral hydrate, propoxyphene napsylate–acetaminophen, zolpidem, and amitriptyline. After 7 years of treatment, on July 31, 2003, her physical function score was 5, pain score 9.9, global score 9.6, and RAPID3 23.5, indicating persistent high severity. In September 2003, she spent a week at a detoxification center, and was weaned off all pain medications. She returned on October 20, 2003, with scores of 0 for functional status, 0.3 for pain, 0.1 for global status, and RAPID3 0.4, indicating near remission status (≤3). She was told she need not return to this clinic. After a typical course for 7 years, an atypical response of a patient with fibromyalgia is documented. (*Courtesy of* Health Report Services. Copyright © 2009 Health Reports Service, Inc. Email: tedpincus@gmail.com.)

Multi-Dimensional Health Assessment Questionnaire (MDHAQ) Scores, Laboratory Tests, Medications
DOB: _Nov 1974_ 1ˢᵗ Visit: _15 Mar 2004_ DX ICD9: _713.1_ Onset: _Jan 2001_ Education: _14_

VISIT DATE	15 Mar 04	24 Mar 04	19 May 04	7 Jun 04	14 Jul 04	15 Aug 05	12 Jul 06
PATIENT SELF-REPORT QUESTIONNAIRE DATA							
FUNCTIONAL STATUS (FN) [0-10]	5.7	7.0	8.0	4.3	0.3	0.3	1.0
PAIN (PN) [0-10]	10	8.5	10	7.2	4.0	1	3.7
GLOBAL STATUS (GL) [0-10]	7.0	8.7	10	7.5	2.0	0	3.1
RAPID3 (0-30)	22.7	24.2	28	19	6.3	1.3	7.8
PHYSICAL MEASURES DATA							
WEIGHT (lbs)	161	156	161	161	160	179	182
BLOOD PRESSURE (mm/Hg)	120/66	122/80	106/70	134/68	112/61	115/78	116/72
LABORATORY DATA							
ESR (mm/hr) [M:0-20 / F:0-30]			76	68	45		
CRP (mg/L) [0-10]			213	65	9		62.8
WBC (thou/uL) [4-11]			9.1	12.7	9.7		11.6
HGB (g/dL) [M:14-18/F:12-16]			10.1	9	9.4		13.3
HCT (%) [M:42-50/F:37-44]			34	31	31		41
PLATELETS (thou/uL) [150-400]			574	475	477		345
ALBUMIN (g/dL) [3.5-5.0]				3.9	4.1		4.3
ALK PHOS (U/L) [40-100]				139	124		92
SGOT (U/L) [4-40]				15	51		17
CREATININE (mg/dL) [0.7-1.5]			0.9	0.8	0.7		0.9
RHEUMATOLOGY MEDICATIONS (C=Change Dose, D=D/C, N=New, O=On at visit, P=Parenteral, R=Resume, S=Short Term, T=Taper)							
Valdecoxib	D-20 QD	O-20 QD	20 QD	D			
Indomethacin SR	N-75 QD	D					
Infliximab		N Q8W	C-6 Q8W	D			
Phenylbutazone		N-100 TID	100 TID	100 TID	D-100 TID		
Adalimumab				N-40 Q2W	40 Q2W	40 Q2W	40 Q2W
Prednisone				D-5 QD		R-3 QD	3 QD
Methotrexate					O-10 QW	15 QWK	15 QWK
Folic Acid					O-1 QD	1 QD	1 QD
Ibuprofen							400 PRN

Fig. 9. Enteropathic arthritis in a 29-year-old man. A 29-year-old man was seen on March 15, 2004, with widespread musculoskeletal pain, most severe in his back. He had a history of ulcerative colitis. On physical examination, he could not reverse his lumbar lordosis, and a radiograph revealed sacroiliitis. He had a score for physical function of 5.7, pain of 10, global status of 7, and RAPID3 of 22.7, indicating high severity (>12). He had been treated with valdecoxib, which was not helpful, and his treatment was changed to indomethacin SR, 75 mg per day. He returned 1 week later with minimal improvement, documented by similar scores for physical function, pain, global status, and RAPID3. He was then treated with phenylbutazone, 100 mg three times a day, which proved only mildly efficacious, because his scores 3 months later, on June 7, 2004, were 4.3 for functional status, 7.2 for pain, 7.5 for global status, and 19 for RAPID3, indicating persistent high severity. At that time he was treated with adalimumab, 40 mg every other week. One month later, his score for physical function was 0.3, pain 4, global status 2, and RAPID3 6.3, indicating moderate severity (6.1–12). Two months later, on August 15, 2005, he had a dramatic response with a reduction of his score for physical function to 0.3, pain to 1, global status to 0, and RAPID3 to 1.3, indicating near remission status (≤3). He has continued this treatment with fluctuating scores for pain. His last recorded visit indicated a RAPID3 score of 7.8, indicating moderate severity (6.1–12), but he is able to work as a store manager effectively. (*Courtesy of* Health Report Services. Copyright © 2009 Health Reports Service, Inc. Email: tedpincus@gmail.com.)

Multi-Dimensional Health Assessment Questionnaire (MDHAQ) Scores, Laboratory Tests, Medications
DOB: _June 1963_ 1ˢᵗ Visit: _26 May 2003_ DX ICD9: _136.10_ Onset: _Jan 1999_ Education: _12_

VISIT DATE	26 May 03	14 Aug 03	12 Nov 03	2 Feb 04	16 Feb 05	10 Aug 05	20 Feb 06
PATIENT SELF-REPORT QUESTIONNAIRE DATA							
FUNCTIONAL STATUS **(FN)** [0-10]	0	0	0	0	0	0	0
PAIN **(PN)** [0-10]	7	0	1	0	0	2.2	0
GLOBAL STATUS **(GL)** [0-10]	5.2	5.1	4.6	0	0	0	0
RAPID3 (0-30)	12.2	5.1	5.6	0	0	2.2	0
PHYSICAL MEASURES DATA							
WEIGHT (lbs)	97	95	102	111.8	120	120	128
BLOOD PRESSURE (mm/Hg)	98/58	122/81	146/64	100/70	114/74	149/91	110/70
LABORATORY DATA							
ESR (mm/hr) [M:0-20 / F:0-30]	15	3	3	3	1	4	1
CRP (mg/L) [0-10]	7	3	0	0	0.4	0.5	0.5
WBC (thou/uL) [4-11]	5.5	8.8	7.4	8.1	6.2	5.5	5.4
HGB (g/dL) [M:14-18/F:12-16]	12.3	13.6	13.4	13.7	14.1	14	12.8
HCT (%) [M:42-50/F:37-44]	35	39	40	41	43	43	40
PLATELETS (thou/uL) [150-400]	432	299	320	316	281	305	324
ALBUMIN (g/dL) [3.5-5.0]	4		4.6	4.4	4.9	4.8	4.4
GLUCOSE (mg/dL) [70-110]	80	89	86	96	97		82
ALK PHOS (U/L) [40-100]	64		53	62	74	63	59
SGOT (U/L) [4-40]	24		27	28	33	33	45
CREATININE (mg/dL) [0.7-1.5]	0.6	0.7	0.6	0.7	0.7		0.7
RHEUMATOLOGY MEDICATIONS (C=Change Dose, D=D/C, N=New, O=On at visit, P=Parenteral, R=Resume, S=Short Term, T=Taper)							
Ibuprofen	O-800 Q6H	800 Q6H					
Colchicine	O-0.6 BID	0.6 BID	0.6 BID	0.6 BID	0.6 BID	0.6 BID	0.6 BID
Prednisone	N-3 QD	C-15 QD	T-8 QD	T-7 QD	C-4 QD	R-3 QD	C-4 QD
Methotrexate		N-10 QW	W-10 QW	W-10 QW	W-10 QW	W-10 QW	W-20 QW
Folic acid				O-1 QD	W-1 QD	W-1 QD	W-1 QD

Fig. 10. Behçet syndrome in a 39-year-old woman. A 39-year-old woman was seen on May 26, 2003, with a history of genital and oral ulcers. A diagnosis of Behçet syndrome had been made by another rheumatologist, who treated her with colchicine, 0.6 mg twice a day, which led to significant improvement, but also led to chronic diarrhea. Her score for physical function was 0, but her score for pain was 7, global status 5.2, and RAPID3 12.2, indicating high severity (>12). Prednisone, 3 mg per day, the usual starting dose in this clinic, was added. She did not have improvement and her dose was raised by her local physician to 15 mg per day, which led to substantial improvement. When she was seen on August 14, 2003, her score for physical function remained at 0, pain had improved from 7 to 0, although global status remained 5.1, and RAPID3 was 5.1, indicating moderate severity (3.1–6). Methotrexate, 10 mg per week, was added, and prednisone was tapered by 1 mg every 2 weeks. Three months later, on November 12, 2003, her prednisone was 8 mg per day; score for physical function remained 0, pain was 1, global status 4.6, and RAPID3 5.6, indicating low severity (3.1–6). Her prednisone tapering schedule was changed to 1 mg every 3 months. On February 16, 2005, scores for function, pain, and global status were all 0, with RAPID3 of 0, indicating near remission (≤3), maintained on 4 mg prednisone per day and 10 mg methotrexate per week. (*Courtesy of* Health Report Services. Copyright © 2009 Health Reports Service, Inc. Email: tedpincus@gmail.com.)

Multi-Dimensional Health Assessment Questionnaire (MDHAQ) Scores, Laboratory Tests, Medications
DOB: _May 1968_ 1ˢᵗ Visit: _22 Sep 2003_ DX ICD9: _579.0_ Onset: _Jan 1971_ Education: _17_

VISIT DATE	22 Sep 03	28 Jan 04	15 Mar 04					
PATIENT SELF-REPORT QUESTIONNAIRE DATA								
FUNCTIONAL STATUS (FN) [0-10]	0	0	0					
PAIN (PN) [0-10]	6.2	7	0					
GLOBAL STATUS (GL) [0-10]	4.5	5.5	0					
RAPID3 (0-30)	10.7	12.5	0					
PHYSICAL MEASURES DATA								
WEIGHT (lbs)	166	169	177					
BLOOD PRESSURE (mm/Hg)	111/84	112/82	130/68					
LABORATORY DATA								
ESR (mm/hr) [M:0-20 / F:0-30]	76		8					
CRP (mg/L) [0-10]	184							
WBC (thou/uL) [4-11]	5		6.5					
HGB (g/dL) [M:14-18/F:12-16]	15.5		15.6					
HCT (%) [M:42-50/F:37-44]	46		47					
PLATELETS (thou/uL) [150-400]	298		232					
ALBUMIN (g/dL) [3.5-5.0]			3.5					
ALK PHOS (U/L) [40-100]			49					
SGOT (U/L) [4-40]			28					
CREATININE (mg/dL) [0.7-1.5]	0.8		1.2					
RHEUMATOLOGY MEDICATIONS (C=Change Dose, D=D/C, N=New, O=On at visit, P=Parenteral, R=Resume, S=Short Term, T=Taper)								
MiraLax	O-17 PRN	17 PRN	17 PRN					
Colchicine		N-0.6 QD	0.6 QD					

Fig. 11. Familial Mediterranean Fever in a 35-year-old man. A 35-year-old man was seen on September 22, 2003. He reported recurrent episodes of abdominal pain since childhood, during which he was bedridden for a day or two, followed by spontaneous recovery. He had received diagnoses of multiple food allergies and gluten enteropathy, but continued to experience attacks of abdominal pain. He had experienced an attack 3 days before the visit. His score for physical function was 0, but pain 6.2, global status 4.5, and RAPID3 10.7, indicating moderate severity (6.1–12). Because of his history of possible allergies and gluten enteropathy, it was elected to analyze his medical records before suggesting any new intervention. His sedimentation rate was 76 mm/h and C-reactive protein 184 mg/dL (upper limit of normal 10) on that date. He returned on January 28, 2004, with scores for physical function of 0, pain 7, global status 5.5, and RAPID3 12.5, indicating high severity (>12). A prescription was given for colchicine, 0.6 mg twice a day. On March 15, 2004, his scores for physical function, pain, global status, and RAPID3 were 0, indicating near remission (≤3). He was then returned to the care of his local physician to manage his colchicine therapy. (*Courtesy of* Health Report Services, 2009.)

a low severity range of less than or equal to 6, or near remission less than or equal to 3, provides reassurance that patient status is satisfactory.

An increase in patient questionnaire scores may result from circumstances other than the rheumatic disease for which the patient is being treated, such as trauma, injury, or acute back pain. This circumstance is similar to an increased erythrocyte sedimentation rate, however, which might be caused by an infection or development of a lymphoma rather than a flare of inflammatory rheumatic disease. All quantitative data must be interpreted by a clinician, along with information from further patient history, physical examination, laboratory tests, and imaging studies, in formulating clinical decisions. Nonetheless, availability of quantitative data can add substantially to the decision process, focus the visit on patient concerns, and document status for comparison at future visits.

The importance of function, pain, global status, and RAPID3 scores remain important considerations in all rheumatic diseases. Inclusion of these scores in a flowsheet that also includes laboratory tests and medications could transform the EMR into a true medical database.

REFERENCES

1. Pincus T, Swearingen C, Wolfe F. Toward a multidimensional health assessment questionnaire (MDHAQ): assessment of advanced activities of daily living and psychological status in the patient friendly health assessment questionnaire format. Arthritis Rheum 1999;42:2220–30.
2. Pincus T, Sokka T, Kautiainen H. Further development of a physical function scale on a multidimensional health assessment questionnaire for standard care of patients with rheumatic diseases. J Rheumatol 2005;32:1432–9.
3. Pincus T, Bergman MJ, Yazici Y, et al. An index of only patient-reported outcome measures, routine assessment of patient index data 3 (RAPID3), in two abatacept clinical trials: similar results to disease activity score (DAS28) and other RAPID indices that include physician-reported measures. Rheumatology (Oxford) 2008; 47:345–9.
4. Pincus T, Swearingen CJ, Bergman M, et al. RAPID3 (routine assessment of patient index data 3), a rheumatoid arthritis index without formal joint counts for routine care: proposed severity categories compared to DAS and CDAI categories. J Rheumatol 2008;35:2136–47.
5. Callahan LF, Pincus T. The P-VAS/D-ADL ratio: a clue from a self-report questionnaire to distinguish rheumatoid arthritis from noninflammatory diffuse musculoskeletal pain. Arthritis Rheum 1990;33:1317–22.
6. DeWalt DA, Reed GW, Pincus T. Further clues to recognition of patients with fibromyalgia from a simple 2-page patient multidimensional health assessment questionnaire (MDHAQ). Clin Exp Rheumatol 2004;22:453–61.

A Standard Protocol to Evaluate Rheumatoid Arthritis (SPERA) for Efficient Capture of Essential Data from a Patient and a Health Professional in a Uniform "Scientific" Format

Theodore Pincus, MD[a],*, Leigh F. Callahan, PhD[b],
Tuulikki Sokka, MD, PhD[c]

KEYWORDS

- Standard protocol to evaluate rheumatoid arthritis (SPERA)
- Questionnaire • Joint count • Database

Rheumatoid arthritis (RA) differs from many chronic diseases, such as hypertension, hypercholesterolemia, and osteoporosis, in that a "gold standard" measure is not available for diagnosis, prognosis and management. Therefore, multiple measures have been assembled into RA classification criteria for enrollment in clinical trials and other clinical research studies, and into indices to assess clinical status. RA indices include measures derived from joint counts, laboratory tests, and a quantitative patient questionnaire. Patient questionnaire data distinguish active from control treatments in clinical trials with relative efficiencies similar to swollen and tender joint counts.[1] Patient questionnaires—not a joint count, radiographic score, or laboratory test—provide the

A version of this article originally appeared in the 21:4 issue of *Best Practice & Research Clinical Rheumatology*.
Supported in part by a research grants from the Arthritis Foundation and the Jack C. Massey Foundation, and EVO-grants of Rheumatism Foundation Hospital, Heinola, Finland.
[a] Division of Rheumatology, Department of Medicine, NYU Hospital for Joint Diseases, New York University School of Medicine, 301 East 17th Street, Room 1608, New York, NY 10003, USA
[b] School of Medicine and Gillings School of Global Public Health, University of North Carolina at Chapel Hill, Chapel Hill, NC, USA
[c] Jyväskylä Central Hospital, Jyväskylä and Medcare Oy, Äänekoski, Finland
* Corresponding author.
E-mail address: tedpincus@gmail.com (T. Pincus).

Rheum Dis Clin N Am 35 (2009) 843–850
doi:10.1016/j.rdc.2009.10.016
0889-857X/09/$ – see front matter © 2009 Elsevier Inc. All rights reserved.

rheumatic.theclinics.com

most significant predictors of all severe long-term outcomes in patients who have RA, including functional status,[2,3] work disability,[4–6] costs,[7] joint replacement surgery,[8] and premature death.[2,9–16] Patient questionnaires provide quantitative data in usual care to assess and document clinical status and guide management.

The value of patient questionnaires in clinical care has led the authors to advocate inclusion of a patient questionnaire at every rheumatology visit. Nonetheless, comprehensive assessment of patients who have RA also requires more than self-report data, from further medical history, physical examination, laboratory tests, imaging studies, and other data. Furthermore, patient self-report is not accurate concerning certain information, such as diagnosis and comorbidities.[17]

Information collected by a physician clearly contributes importantly to management decisions. Most of this information is not collected according to a uniform format, even at baseline for clinical trials and other clinical research, much less in usual clinical care. For example, comorbidities generally are more common in patients who have RA than in the general population,[18] and are a significant predictor of mortality in RA, at higher levels than radiographic scores or laboratory tests.[13,16] Data concerning comorbidities in patients who have RA are collected with relatively similar lists in clinical trials and clinical care, but in different formats, so it is difficult to pool data into multicenter databases for clinical research.

The value of a standard format on a patient questionnaire suggests that important information collected by the physician could also be collected in a standard format. A physician global estimate of patient status, assess on a 10-cm visual analog scale (VAS), and a formal quantitative joint count are performed according to standard formats. Collection of other physician/assessor information that usually is collected in patients with RA–concerning classification criteria, family history, extra-articular disease, comorbidities, and joint surgeries–in a standard format could improve clinical care and assessment of quality, and be informative in clinical research.

Over the past 2 decades, the authors have used a three-page standard format for efficient collection of data in patients who have inflammatory arthritis, termed a *standard protocol to evaluate rheumatoid arthritis* (SPERA).[19,20] This format has proven useful for collecting data in many studies evaluating prognosis and monitoring of patients. SPERA has contributed to the development of a 28-joint count[21]; observation of radiographic damage in most patients within the first 2 years of disease[22]; recognition that patient questionnaires are correlated significantly with joint counts, radiographic scores, and laboratory tests,[23] while providing more significant predictors of work disability[4] and mortality[11,13] than traditional measures; and observations that a small proportion of patients were eligible for clinical trials in contemporary care of RA.[24,25] The SPERA format helped show that all patients who had RA seen by the senior author in 2000 had considerably better status than all patients seen in 1985 in the same clinical setting.[26] SPERA has been used to collect comprehensive baseline clinical data in 8039 patients in 32 countries for the Quantitative Standard Monitoring of Patients with Rheumatoid Arthritis (QUEST-RA) program.[27–29]

SPERA includes data from patients and clinicians. Patients complete a standard self-report questionnaire—a health assessment questionnaire (HAQ),[30] multidimensional HAQ (MDHAQ),[31,32] or variant, including a four-page format used for QUEST-RA. The clinician completes a three-page form (**Figs. 1–3**), which addresses:

1. Clinical features, including onset of RA, classification criteria, extra-articular disease, comorbidities, and surgeries (see **Fig. 1**);
2. Medications taken for RA (see **Fig. 2**); and

R663-QUEST-RA -CLUE   **Clinical Lifetime Updateable Evaluation (CLUE – MED)**
Rheumatoid Arthritis Clinical Features

ID _____ SITE _____ Date of Birth _____ Today's date _____
(day/month/year)   (day/month/year)

CLUE FORM COMPLETED BY _____   Rheumatologist _____

HISTORY OF ONSET OF RA:

RA-1st Symptoms (Mo/Yr) _____

RA-Diagnosis (Mo/Yr) _____

What was 1st DMARD(s) _____

1st DMARD (Mo/Yr) _____

COMORBIDITIES:	Ever? "—" or "+"	If "+" Mo/Yr
Hypertension	_____	_____
Angina	_____	_____
Heart Attack	_____	_____
Coronary Artery Disease	_____	_____
Other Heart Disease	_____	_____
Hyperlipidemia	_____	_____
Peripheral Vascular Disease	_____	_____
Peptic Ulcer	_____	_____
Inflammatory Bowel Disease	_____	_____
Impaired Renal Function	_____	_____
Asthma	_____	_____
Chronic Bronchitis	_____	_____
Diabetes Mellitus	_____	_____
Thyroid Disease	_____	_____
Cancer	_____	_____
Stroke	_____	_____
Parkinson's Disease	_____	_____
Chronic Back Pain	_____	_____
Musculoskeletal Trauma	_____	_____
Low Energy Fractures	_____	_____
Osteoporosis At Scan	_____	_____
Osteoarthritis	_____	_____
Infection Requiring Hospitalization	_____	_____
Herpes Zoster/Shingles	_____	_____
Fibromyalgia	_____	_____
Psoriasis	_____	_____
Cataracts	_____	_____
Psychiatric Disease	_____	_____
AIDS	_____	_____
Alcoholism	_____	_____

ARA CRITERIA FOR RA:

	Ever? "—" or "+"	If "+", Mo/Yr
Morning Stiffness > 1 hour	_____	_____
Soft tissue swelling of >= 3 Joint Groups	_____	_____
Swelling of PIP, MCP, or Wrist Joints	_____	_____
Symmetrical Swelling	_____	_____
Subcutaneous Nodule	_____	_____
Positive Rheumatoid Factor	_____	_____
Highest Rheumatoid Factor	_____	
Radiographic Erosion	_____	_____

EXTRA-ARTICULAR DISEASE:

	Ever? "—" or "+"	Onset Mo/Yr
Pulmonary Fibrosis	_____	_____
Pulmonary Nodules	_____	_____
Clinical Pericarditis	_____	_____
Felty's Syndrome	_____	_____
Lymphadenopathy	_____	_____
Carpal Tunnel	_____	_____
Tarsal Tunnel	_____	_____
Vasculitis	_____	_____
Scleritis	_____	_____
Neuropathy	_____	_____
Raynaud's phenomenon	_____	_____
Dry Eyes	_____	_____
Dry Mouth	_____	_____

RADIOGRAPH DATE (PA hands & wrists and feet; Mo/Yr):
_____

SURGERIES:	Ever? "—" or "+"	If "+", Mo/Yr	Mo/Yr	Mo/Yr:
Carpal Tunnel	_____	_____	_____	_____
Heart Bypass	_____	_____	_____	_____
Back Surgery	_____	_____	_____	_____
Cataract	_____	_____	_____	_____

JT SURGERY/FRACTURE:
(A-Arthroscopy, S-Synovectomy, TJR-Replacement,
JF-Fusion, JR-Reconstruction, F-Fracture)
R/L Hand(mo/yr)_____R/L Elbow(mo/yr)_____
R/L Hip(mo/yr)_____R/L Foot(mo/yr)_____
R/L Knee(mo/yr)_____C-Spine(mo/yr)_____

Fig. 1. Clinical Lifetime Updateable Evaluation form for clinical features of rheumatoid arthritis—onset features, classification criteria, extra-articular disease, comorbidities, surgeries.

3. A 42-joint count, which includes 10 proximal interphalangeal (PIP) joints of the hand, 10 metacarpophalangeal joints, 2 wrists, 2 elbows, 2 shoulders, 2 hips, 2 knees, 2 ankles, and 10 metatarsophalangeal joints (hips and shoulders are not scored for swelling). All joints are scored for tenderness, swelling (except hips and shoulders), limited motion, and surgery, with a space to indicate that a joint is normal (see **Fig. 3**).

The first two pages of the physician-provided data in SPERA are designated as Clinical Lifetime Updateable Evaluation (CLUE) forms. They are designed to indicate

R663-QUEST-RA -CLUE   **Clinical Lifetime Updateable Evaluation (CLUE – MED)**
                                                  Rheumatoid Arthritis Medications

ID _____ SITE _____ Date of Birth _____ Today's date _____
                                                                    (day/month/year)   (day/month/year)

Please record ALL pills taken by the patient over the last TWO WEEKS, with or without a prescription. Please include aspirin
birth control pills, pain pills, alternative therapies, health supplements and any pills sold in health food stores:

NAME OF DRUG, MEDICINE OR ALTERNATIVE THERAPY	DOSE (if known)	How Many per day or week?	NAME OF DRUG, MEDICINE OR ALTERNATIVE THERAPY	DOSE (if known)	How Many Per day or week?
1.			11.		
2.			12.		
3.			13.		
4.			14.		
5.			15.		
6.			16.		
7.			17.		
8.			18.		
9.			19.		
10.			20.		

DMARD Review

	Ever −/+	Start date (mo/yr)	Stop date (mo/yr)	Takes Now −/+	How Many Years Taken optional	Toxicities Describe toxicities or record NONE if no toxicities	Reason to Discontinue N=No efficacy T=Toxicity (please list) L= Loss of efficacy O=Other (please list)
PREDNISONE						Approx daily dose:	
METHOTREXATE							
HYDROXYCHLOROQUINE							
SULFASALAZINE							
CYCLOSPORINE							
AZATHIOPRINE							
LEFLUNOMIDE							
ETANERCEPT							
INFLIXIMAB							
ANAKINRA							
ADALIMUMAB							
RITUXIMAB							
ABATACEPT							
CERTOLIZUMAB							

Additional drugs and/or other courses may be entered in blank spaces.

Fig. 2. Clinical Lifetime Updateable Evaluation form for medications taken for rheumatoid arthritis.

a negative response by a "−," which may then be amended to a "+," and may be kept in a designated position in a patient's record, generally on color-coded paper, for updating in standard care. One additional document, a radiographic scoring sheet, may be included for a comprehensive baseline database for patients. These forms could also serve as templates for electronic medical records.

Software is available to record and manage these data. The SPERA protocol captures the most important baseline information a clinician wishes to know about a patient who might have RA, in 15 to 20 minutes or less, to provide baseline information for a clinical trial, observational research study, or usual clinical care. The protocol helps avoid collection of extensive information that may be of limited or no value but

R663-QUEST-RA -CLUE   **Clinical Lifetime Updateable Evaluation (CLUE – JC)**
                                                            Joint Count Examination

ID _____ SITE _____ Date of Birth _____ Today's date _____
                                                        (day/month/year)   (day/month/year)

Please record the current results of laboratory tests for:

ESR _____ CRP _____ (ref. values: _____)
Hemoglobin _____ Rheumatoid Factor _____ (ref. values: _____)

Please mark below your assessment of the patient's current disease activity:

NO
ACTIVITY ├──┤ VERY
                                                                                                 ACTIVE

JOINT COUNT - SCORE EACH JOINT AS: "+" for **positive or abnormal** versus "- " for **negative or normal**

	If NORM, mark"-" & go to next joint	Tender or pain on motion	Swollen	Limited motion or deformed	# Surger-ies§		If NORM, mark"-" & go to next joint	Tender or pain on motion	Swollen	Limited motion or deformed	# Surger-ies§
R-PIP1	__	__	__	__	__	L-PIP1	__	__	__	__	__
R-PIP2	__	__	__	__	__	L-PIP2	__	__	__	__	__
R-PIP3	__	__	__	__	__	L-PIP3	__	__	__	__	__
R-PIP4	__	__	__	__	__	L-PIP4	__	__	__	__	__
R-PIP5	__	__	__	__	__	L-PIP5	__	__	__	__	__
R-MCP1	__	__	__	__	__	L-MCP1	__	__	__	__	__
R-MCP2	__	__	__	__	__	L-MCP2	__	__	__	__	__
R-MCP3	__	__	__	__	__	L-MCP3	__	__	__	__	__
R-MCP4	__	__	__	__	__	L-MCP4	__	__	__	__	__
R-MCP5	__	__	__	__	__	L-MCP5	__	__	__	__	__
R-WRIST	__	__	__	__	__	L-WRIST	__	__	__	__	__
R-ELBOW	__	__	__	__	__	L-ELBOW	__	__	__	__	__
R-SHLDR	__	__	XXX	__	__	L-SHLDR	__	__	XXX	__	__
R-HIP	__	__	XXX	__	__	L-HIP	__	__	XXX	__	__
R-KNEE	__	__	__	__	__	L-KNEE	__	__	__	__	__
R-ANKLE	__	__	__	__	__	L-ANKLE	__	__	__	__	__
R-MTP1	__	__	__	__	__	L-MTP1	__	__	__	__	__
R-MTP2	__	__	__	__	__	L-MTP2	__	__	__	__	__
R-MTP3	__	__	__	__	__	L-MTP3	__	__	__	__	__
R-MTP4	__	__	__	__	__	L-MTP4	__	__	__	__	__
R-MTP5	__	__	__	__	__	L-MTP5	__	__	__	__	__

§ - **S** = Synovectomy **J** = Total Joint Replacement (TJR) **O** = Other

Description only - not in formal joint count:

NECK __ _____
BACK __ _____

Fig. 3. A 42-joint count, which includes 10 proximal interphalangeal (PIP) joints of the hand, 10 metacarpophalangeal joints, 2 wrists, 2 elbows, 2 shoulders, 2 hips, 2 knees, 2 ankles, and 10 metatarsophalangeal joints (hips and shoulders are not scored for swelling). All joints are scored for tenderness, swelling (except hips and shoulders), limited motion, and surgery, with a dash to indicate that a joint is normal.

that may add expense, time, and effort for patients and health professionals. However, the SPERA does not preclude collection of additional data for specialized studies.

This SPERA format is not advocated as optimal, but is presented as an example of a possible approach to a standard format for collection of information in a standard format by the rheumatology community. A standard uniform format requires consensus from various rheumatology centers, extending the concept of a uniform clinical database for rheumatic diseases proposed by Fries[33,34] in the 1970s. A database such as the SPERA could be used at baseline for all clinical trials and in standard care to facilitate analyses of long-term outcomes of rheumatic diseases.

SPERA incorporates the five core domains listed in a consensus for long-term observational studies from an Outcome Measures in Rheumatoid Arthritis Clinical Trials (OMERACT) conference in 1998: health status, disease process, damage, mortality, and toxicity/adverse reactions.[35] A consensus on a uniform standardized assessment methodology among various rheumatology centers would seem desirable. A similar format could be incorporated into clinical trials and long-term observational research, so the clinical trial could provide baseline information for observation of long-term outcomes, similar and available for pooled comparisons from all clinical trials.

A standard format to list comorbidities could function like an erythrocyte sedimentation rate (ESR) or pain visual analog scale to facilitate comparisons in different clinical settings or different countries with different treatments over time. Although several scales are available to assess comorbidities,[36–39] these scales are not used widely in rheumatology clinical research or standard clinical care. These data could enhance analyses of questions, such as whether therapy with biological agents might reduce the prevalence of subsequent long term comorbidities.

The process of recording data in a standardized uniform format may seem to require considerable extra time on the part of the rheumatologist and to detract from efficiency in clinical care. Ironically, with very brief experience, the opposite is generally true. A standardized format in clinical care can provide information at a glance, which otherwise may take 10 to 100 times as long to collect, as seen with patient questionnaire data concerning physical function, pain, or global status on the MDHAQ. A standard format for comorbidities and medications could have a similar benefit.

REFERENCES

1. Tugwell P, Wells G, Strand V, et al. Clinical improvement as reflected in measures of function and health-related quality of life following treatment with leflunomide compared with methotrexate in patients with rheumatoid arthritis: sensitivity and relative efficiency to detect a treatment effect in a twelve-month, placebo-controlled trial. Leflunomide rheumatoid arthritis investigators group. Arthritis Rheum 2000;43:506–14.
2. Pincus T, Callahan LF, Sale WG, et al. Severe functional declines, work disability, and increased mortality in seventy-five rheumatoid arthritis patients studied over nine years. Arthritis Rheum 1984;27:864–72.
3. Wolfe F, Cathey MA. The assessment and prediction of functional disability in rheumatoid arthritis. J Rheumatol 1991;18:1298–306.
4. Callahan LF, Bloch DA, Pincus T. Identification of work disability in rheumatoid arthritis: physical, radiographic and laboratory variables do not add explanatory power to demographic and functional variables. J Clin Epidemiol 1992;45: 127–38.
5. Wolfe F, Hawley DJ. The longterm outcomes of rheumatoid arthritis: work disability: a prospective 18 year study of 823 patients. J Rheumatol 1998;25: 2108–17.
6. Sokka T, Kautiainen H, Möttönen T, et al. Work disability in rheumatoid arthritis 10 years after the diagnosis. J Rheumatol 1999;26:1681–5.
7. Lubeck DP, Spitz PW, Fries JF, et al. A multicenter study of annual health service utilization and costs in rheumatoid arthritis. Arthritis Rheum 1986;29:488–93.
8. Wolfe F, Zwillich SH. The long-term outcomes of rheumatoid arthritis: a 23-year prospective, longitudinal study of total joint replacement and its predictors in 1,600 patients with rheumatoid arthritis. Arthritis Rheum 1998;41:1072–82.

9. Wolfe F, Kleinheksel SM, Cathey MA, et al. The clinical value of the Stanford Health Assessment Questionnaire Functional Disability Index in patients with rheumatoid arthritis. J Rheumatol 1988;15:1480–8.
10. Leigh JP, Fries JF. Mortality predictors among 263 patients with rheumatoid arthritis. J Rheumatol 1991;18:1307–12.
11. Pincus T, Brooks RH, Callahan LF. Prediction of long-term mortality in patients with rheumatoid arthritis according to simple questionnaire and joint count measures. Ann Intern Med 1994;120:26–34.
12. Callahan LF, Cordray DS, Wells G, et al. Formal education and five-year mortality in rheumatoid arthritis: mediation by helplessness scale scores. Arthritis Care Res 1996;9:463–72.
13. Callahan LF, Pincus T, Huston JW III, et al. Measures of activity and damage in rheumatoid arthritis: depiction of changes and prediction of mortality over five years. Arthritis Care Res 1997;10:381–94.
14. Söderlin MK, Nieminen P, Hakala M. Functional status predicts mortality in a community based rheumatoid arthritis population. J Rheumatol 1998;25:1895–9.
15. Sokka T, Hakkinen A, Krishnan E, et al. Similar prediction of mortality by the health assessment questionnaire in patients with rheumatoid arthritis and the general population. Ann Rheum Dis 2004;63:494–7.
16. Sokka T, Abelson B, Pincus T. Mortality in rheumatoid arthritis: 2008 update. Clin Exp Rheumatol 2008;26:S35–61.
17. Kvien TK, Glennås A, Knudsrod OG, et al. The validity of self-reported diagnosis of rheumatoid arthritis: results from a population survey followed by clinical examinations. J Rheumatol 1996;23:1866–71.
18. Mitchell JM, Burkhauser RV, Pincus T. The importance of age, education, and co-morbidity in the substantial earnings losses of individuals with symmetric polyarthritis. Arthritis Rheum 1988;31:348–57.
19. Pincus T, Brooks RH, Callahan LF. A proposed standard protocol to evaluate rheumatoid arthritis (SPERA) that includes measures of inflammatory activity, joint damage, and longterm outcomes. J Relig 1999;26:473–80.
20. Pincus T, Sokka T. A three-page Standard Protocol to Evaluate Rheumatoid Arthritis (SPERA) for efficient capture of essential data from patients and health professionals in standard clinical care and clinical research. Best Pract Res Clin Rheumatol 2007;21:677–85.
21. Fuchs HA, Brooks RH, Callahan LF, et al. A simplified twenty-eight joint quantitative articular index in rheumatoid arthritis. Arthritis Rheum 1989;32:531–7.
22. Fuchs HA, Kaye JJ, Callahan LF, et al. Evidence of significant radiographic damage in rheumatoid arthritis within the first 2 years of disease. J Rheumatol 1989;16:585–91.
23. Pincus T, Callahan LF, Brooks RH, et al. Self-report questionnaire scores in rheumatoid arthritis compared with traditional physical, radiographic, and laboratory measures. Ann Intern Med 1989;110:259–66.
24. Sokka T, Pincus T. Most patients receiving routine care for rheumatoid arthritis in 2001 did not meet inclusion criteria for most recent clinical trials or American College of Rheumatology criteria for remission. J Rheumatol 2003;30:1138–46.
25. Sokka T, Pincus T. Eligibility of patients in routine care for major clinical trials of anti-tumor necrosis factor alpha agents in rheumatoid arthritis. Arthritis Rheum 2003;48:313–8.
26. Pincus T, Sokka T, Kautiainen H. Further development of a physical function scale on a multidimensional health assessment questionnaire for standard care of patients with rheumatic diseases. J Rheumatol 2005;32:1432–9.

27. Sokka T, Kautiainen H, Toloza S, et al. QUEST-RA: quantitative clinical assessment of patients with rheumatoid arthritis seen in standard rheumatology care in 15 countries. Ann Rheum Dis 2007;66:1491–6.

28. Sokka T, Toloza S, Cutolo M, et al. Women, men, and rheumatoid arthritis: analyses of disease activity, disease characteristics, and treatments in the QUEST-RA Study. Arthritis Res Ther 2009;11:R7.

29. Sokka T, Kautiainen H, Pincus T, et al. Disparities in rheumatoid arthritis disease activity according to gross domestic product in 25 countries in the QUEST-RA database. Ann Rheum Dis 2009;68:1666–72.

30. Fries JF, Spitz P, Kraines RG, et al. Measurement of patient outcome in arthritis. Arthritis Rheum 1980;23:137–45.

31. Pincus T, Bergman MJ, Yazici Y, et al. An index of only patient-reported outcome measures, routine assessment of patient index data 3 (RAPID3), in two abatacept clinical trials: similar results to disease activity score (DAS28) and other RAPID indices that include physician-reported measures. Rheumatology (Oxford) 2008;47:345–9.

32. Pincus T, Swearingen CJ, Bergman M, et al. RAPID3 (routine assessment of patient index data 3), a rheumatoid arthritis index without formal joint counts for routine care: proposed severity categories compared to DAS and CDAI categories. J Rheumatol 2008;35:2136–47.

33. Fries JF. Time-oriented patient records and a computer databank. JAMA 1972; 222:1536–42.

34. Fries JF. Editorial: a data bank for the clinician? N Engl J Med 1976;294:1400–2.

35. Wolfe F, Lassere M, van der Heijde D, et al. Preliminary core set of domains and reporting requirements for longitudinal observational studies in rheumatology. J Rheumatol 1999;26:484–9.

36. Parkerson GR Jr, Broadhead WE, Tse CKJ. The Duke Severity of Illness Checklist (DUSOI) for measurement of severity and comorbidity. J Clin Epidemiol 1993;46: 379–93.

37. Katz JN, Chang LC, Sangha O, et al. Can comorbidity be measured by questionnaire rather than medical record review? Med Care 1996;34:73–84.

38. Cleves MA, Sanchez N, Draheim M. Evaluation of two competing methods for calculating Charlson's comorbidity index when analyzing short-term mortality using administrative data. J Clin Epidemiol 1997;50:903–8.

39. Charlson ME, Pompei P, Ales KL, et al. A new method of classifying prognostic comorbidity in longitudinal studies: development and validation. J Chronic Dis 1987;40:373–83.

Quality Control of a Medical History: Improving Accuracy with Patient Participation, Supported by a Four-Page Version of the Multidimensional Health Assessment Questionnaire (MDHAQ)

Theodore Pincus, MD[a],*, Yusuf Yazici, MD[a],
Christopher J. Swearingen, PhD[b]

KEYWORDS

- Medical history • Medical record
- Multidimensional health assessment questionnaire (MDHAQ)
- Quality control

Information in the medical records of many patients may be missing, incomplete, or inaccurate. Many omissions and errors are innocuous (eg, missing information concerning an appendectomy or distant hospitalization for pneumonia, or recording of an event as occurring in 1984 rather than 1994). Serious errors may be seen in many medical records, however, such as omission of allergies to medications,

Supported in part by grants from the Arthritis Foundation, the Jack C. Massey Foundation, Bristol-Myers Squibb, and Amgen.

A version of this article originally appeared in the 21:4 issue of *Best Practice & Research: Clinical Rheumatology*.

[a] Division of Rheumatology, Department of Medicine, New York University School of Medicine and NYU Hospital for Joint Diseases, Room 1608, 301 East 17th Street, New York, NY 10003, USA
[b] Department of Pediatrics, Biostatistics Program, University of Arkansas for Medical Sciences, Little Rock, AR, USA
* Corresponding author.
E-mail address: tedpincus@gmail.com (T. Pincus).

Rheum Dis Clin N Am 35 (2009) 851–860
doi:10.1016/j.rdc.2009.10.014
0889-857X/09/$ – see front matter © 2009 Elsevier Inc. All rights reserved.

rheumatic.theclinics.com

Multi-Dimensional Health Assessment Questionnaire (R811-NP4)

This questionnaire includes information not available from blood tests, X-rays, or any source other than you. Please try to answer each question, even if you do not think it is related to you at this time. Try to complete as much as you can yourself, but if you need help, please ask. <u>There are no right or wrong answers.</u> Please answer exactly as you think or feel. Thank you.

1. Please check (√) the ONE best answer for your abilities at this time:

OVER THE LAST WEEK, were you able to:	Without ANY Difficulty	With SOME Difficulty	With MUCH Difficulty	UNABLE To Do
a. Dress yourself, including tying shoelaces and doing buttons?	0	1	2	3
b. Get in and out of bed?	0	1	2	3
c. Lift a full cup or glass to your mouth?	0	1	2	3
d. Walk outdoors on flat ground?	0	1	2	3
e. Wash and dry your entire body?	0	1	2	3
f. Bend down to pick up clothing from the floor?	0	1	2	3
g. Turn regular faucets on and off?	0	1	2	3
h. Get in and out of a car, bus, train, or airplane?	0	1	2	3
i. Walk two miles or three kilometers, if you wish?	0	1	2	3
j. Participate in recreational activities and sports as you would like, if you wish?	0	1	2	3
k. Get a good night's sleep?	0	1.1	2.2	3.3
l. Deal with feelings of anxiety or being nervous?	0	1.1	2.2	3.3
m. Deal with feelings of depression or feeling blue?	0	1.1	2.2	3.3

FOR OFFICE USE ONLY

1.a† FN (0-10): ☐

1=0.3   16=5.3
2=0.7   17=5.7
3=1.0   18=6.0
4=1.3   19=6.3
5=1.7   20=6.7
6=2.0   21=7.0
7=2.3   22=7.3
8=2.7   23=7.7
9=3.0   24=8.0
10=3.3   25=8.3
11=3.7   26=8.7
12=4.0   27=9.0
13=4.3   28=9.3
14=4.7   29=9.7
15=5.0   30=10

2.PN (0-10): ☐

2. How much pain have you had because of your condition OVER THE PAST WEEK? Please indicate below how severe your pain has been:

NO PAIN ○ PAIN AS BAD AS IT COULD BE
0   0.5   1.0   1.5   2.0   2.5   3.0   3.5   4.0   4.5   5.0   5.5   6.0   6.5   7.0   7.5   8.0   8.5   9.0   9.5   10

4.PTGL (0-10): ☐

RAPID 3 (0-30) ☐

3. Please place a check (√) in the appropriate spot to indicate the amount of pain you are having today in each of the joint areas listed below:

	None	Mild	Moderate	Severe		None	Mild	Moderate	Severe
a. LEFT FINGERS	☐0	☐1	☐2	☐3	i. RIGHT FINGERS	☐0	☐1	☐2	☐3
b. LEFT WRIST	☐0	☐1	☐2	☐3	j. RIGHT WRIST	☐0	☐1	☐2	☐3
c. LEFT ELBOW	☐0	☐1	☐2	☐3	k. RIGHT ELBOW	☐0	☐1	☐2	☐3
d. LEFT SHOULDER	☐0	☐1	☐2	☐3	l. RIGHT SHOULDER	☐0	☐1	☐2	☐3
e. LEFT HIP	☐0	☐1	☐2	☐3	m. RIGHT HIP	☐0	☐1	☐2	☐3
f. LEFT KNEE	☐0	☐1	☐2	☐3	n. RIGHT KNEE	☐0	☐1	☐2	☐3
g. LEFT ANKLE	☐0	☐1	☐2	☐3	o. RIGHT ANKLE	☐0	☐1	☐2	☐3
h. LEFT TOES	☐0	☐1	☐2	☐3	p. RIGHT TOES	☐0	☐1	☐2	☐3
q. NECK	☐0	☐1	☐2	☐3	r. BACK	☐0	☐1	☐2	☐3

Cat:
HS = >12
MS = 6.1-12
LS = 3.1-6
R = <3

4. Considering all the ways in which illness and health conditions may affect you at this time, please indicate below how you are doing:

VERY WELL ○ VERY POORLY
0   0.5   1.0   1.5   2.0   2.5   3.0   3.5   4.0   4.5   5.0   5.5   6.0   6.5   7.0   7.5   8.0   8.5   9.0   9.5   10

Please turn to the other side

Copyright: Health Report Services, Telephone 615-479-5303, E-mail tedpincus@gmail.com

Fig. 1. A four-page (two sheets of paper) version of the MDHAQ designed for the initial visit. (*Courtesy of* Health Report Services, Copyright © 2009 Health Reports Service, Inc. Email: tedpincus@gmail.com.)

incorrect dosage of prescribed medications, and errors concerning relevant severe comorbidities.

Patient self-report questionnaires and simple computerized databases provide an opportunity for improved quality control of the patient history in a medical record. The primary innovation involves review of the available history by the patient as a partner in the infrastructure of usual medical care. This method has been implemented by the senior author since 2000 using Microsoft Access software, improving

5. Please check (√) if you have experienced any of the following <u>over the last month:</u>

__Fever	__Lump in your throat	__Paralysis of arms or legs	**FOR OFFICE USE ONLY**
__Weight gain (>10 lbs)	__Cough	__Numbness or tingling of arms or legs	
__Weight loss (>10 lbs)	__Shortness of breath	__Fainting spells	**5. ROS:**
__Feeling sickly	__Wheezing	__Swelling of hands	
__Headaches	__Pain in the chest	__Swelling of ankles	
__Unusual fatigue	__Heart pounding (palpitations)	__Swelling in other joints	
__Swollen glands	__Trouble swallowing	__Joint pain	
__Loss of appetite	__Heartburn or stomach gas	__Back pain	
__Skin rash or hives	__Stomach pain or cramps	__Neck pain	
__Unusual bruising or bleeding	__Nausea	__Use of drugs not sold in stores	
__Other skin problems	__Vomiting	__Smoking cigarettes	
__Loss of hair	__Constipation	__More than 2 alcoholic drinks per day	
__Dry eyes	__Diarrhea	__Depression - feeling blue	
__Other eye problems	__Dark or bloody stools	__Anxiety - feeling nervous	
__Problems with hearing	__Problems with urination	__Problems with thinking	
__Ringing in the ears	__Gynecological (female) problems	__Problems with memory	
__Stuffy nose	__Dizziness	__Problems with sleeping	
__Sores in the mouth	__Losing your balance	__Sexual problems	
__Dry mouth	__Muscle pain, aches, or cramps	__Burning in sex organs	
__Problems with smell or taste	__Muscle weakness	__Problems with social activities	

Please check (√) here if you have had none of the above over the last month: _____.

6. When you awakened in the morning OVER THE LAST WEEK, did you feel stiff? ☐ No   ☐ Yes
If "No," please go to Item 7. If "**Yes**," please indicate the number of minutes_____, or hours _____ until you are as limber as you will be for the day.

7. How do you feel TODAY compared to ONE WEEK AGO? Please check (✓) only one.
Much Better ☐ (1),   Better ☐ (2),   the Same ☐ (3),   Worse ☐ (4),   Much Worse ☐ (5) than one week ago

8. How often do you exercise aerobically (sweating, increased heart rate, shortness of breath) **for at least one-half hour** (30 minutes)? **Please check (✓) only one.**

☐ 3 or more times a week (3)   ☐ 1-2 times per month (1)
☐ 1-2 times per week   (2)   ☐ Do not exercise regularly (0)   ☐ Cannot exercise due to disability/ handicap (9)

9. How much of a problem has UNUSUAL fatigue or tiredness been for you OVER THE PAST WEEK?

FATIGUE IS   ○   FATIGUE IS A
NO PROBLEM   0 0.5 1.0 1.5 2.0 2.5 3.0 3.5 4.0 4.5 5.0 5.5 6.0 6.5 7.0 7.5 8.0 8.5 9.0 9.5 10   MAJOR PROBLEM

10. Over the last 6 months have you had: [Please check (√)]

☐No ☐Yes An operation or new illness	☐No ☐Yes Change(s) of arthritis or other medication
☐No ☐Yes Medical emergency or stay overnight in hospital	☐No ☐Yes Change(s) of address
☐No ☐Yes A fall, broken bone, or other accident or trauma	☐No ☐Yes Change(s) of marital status
☐No ☐Yes An important new symptom or medical problem	☐No ☐Yes Change job or work duties, quit work, retired
☐No ☐Yes Side effect(s) of any medication or drug	☐No ☐Yes Change of medical insurance, Medicare, etc.
☐No ☐Yes Smoke cigarettes regularly	☐No ☐Yes Change of primary care or other doctor

Please explain any "Yes" answer below, or indicate any other health matter that affects you:

_____

_____

11. Please list below any medications which you cannot take because you are allergic to them:

_____   _____   _____   _____

12. Please list below anything else (grass, molds, pollens, etc.) you might be allergic to:

_____   _____   _____   _____

Fig. 1. (continued)

accuracy of the medical record with minimal professional effort, while saving time for the physician.

Five simple steps that differ from usual procedures to collect a medical history are the basis for this approach to quality control of the patient history in the medical record.

STEP 1: THE PATIENT COMPLETES A FOUR-PAGE VERSION OF THE MULTIDIMENSIONAL HEALTH ASSESSMENT QUESTIONNAIRE AT THE INITIAL VISIT

The multidimensional health assessment questionnaire (MDHAQ) is informative for any patient with a rheumatic (or any) disease. The basic MDHAQ includes two sides of

13. Please check (✓) either "No" or "Yes" to indicate whether or not you have any of the conditions below:
    Have you ever had: If you answer "Yes", please list AGE or YEAR when it began.
                                    AGE or YEAR   **AGE or YEAR**

High Blood Pressure or				Gynecological (Female)/		
Hypertension	__No	__Yes	___ or ___	Prostate (Male) problem	__No __Yes	___ or ___
Heart attack	__No	__Yes	___ or ___	Severe allergies	__No __Yes	___ or ___
Other heart disease	__No	__Yes	___ or ___	Rheumatoid arthritis	__No __Yes	___ or ___
Cancer	__No	__Yes	___ or ___	Osteoarthritis	__No __Yes	___ or ___
Stroke	__No	__Yes	___ or ___	Lupus	__No __Yes	___ or ___
Bronchitis or Emphysema	__No	__Yes	___ or ___	Back or spine problems	__No __Yes	___ or ___
Asthma	__No	__Yes	___ or ___	Fibromyalgia (Fibrositis)	__No __Yes	___ or ___
Other Lung problem	__No	__Yes	___ or ___	Osteoporosis	__No __Yes	___ or ___
Anemia (Low Blood)	__No	__Yes	___ or ___	Broken bones after age 50	__No __Yes	___ or ___
Other hematologic problem	__No	__Yes	___ or ___	Dry mouth	__No __Yes	___ or ___
Stomach ulcer	__No	__Yes	___ or ___	Dry eyes	__No __Yes	___ or ___
Other gastrointestinal				Cataracts	__No __Yes	___ or ___
(GI) problem	__No	__Yes	___ or ___	Parkinson's disease	__No __Yes	___ or ___
Thyroid problem	__No	__Yes	___ or ___	Depression	__No __Yes	___ or ___
Diabetes	__No	__Yes	___ or ___	Mental illness	__No __Yes	___ or ___
Kidney problem	__No	__Yes	___ or ___	Alcoholism	__No __Yes	___ or ___

Other _____ ___ or ___   Other _____ ___ or ___
        (Please name)   (Please name)

14. Please list below all operations you have ever had. Please check (✓) here if none: _____.
             Operation   Year   Surgeon   Hospital, City, State
1. _____ _____ _____ _____
2. _____ _____ _____ _____
3. _____ _____ _____ _____
4. _____ _____ _____ _____
                           (You may continue below or on a separate page)

15. Please list below all major illnesses or hospital admissions (other than for operations).
    Please check (✓) here if none: _____.
    Illness or Reason for hospitalization   Year   Hospital, City, State
1. _____ _____ _____
2. _____ _____ _____
3. _____ _____ _____
4. _____ _____ _____
                           (You may continue below or on a separate page)

16. The questions below concern your family medical history:
                        If Living   **If Deceased**
            Birth Year or Age   Any Major Medical Conditions   Year or Age at death   Cause(s) of death

Father	_____	_____	_____	_____
Mother	_____	_____	_____	_____
Brother(s)	_____	_____	_____	_____
Sister(s)	_____	_____	_____	_____
Son(s)	_____	_____	_____	_____
Daughter(s)	_____	_____	_____	_____

17. Any blood relative (parent, child, brother, sister, aunt, uncle) with: If "Yes", give relationship.
                        No   Yes   ____ Relation(s) ____   No   Yes   ____ Relation(s) ____
Rheumatoid Arthritis   ___   ___   _____   Lupus or SLE   ___   ___   _____

18. Any illnesses which run in the family? _____

Copyright: Health Report Services, Telephone 615-470-5303, E-mail tedpincus@gmail.com

Fig. 1. (*continued*)

a single sheet of paper, with scales for physical function, pain, global status, and fatigue; a self-report joint count; review of systems; recent medical history; queries about exercise, change in status, and morning stiffness; and demographic data.

A four-page (two sheets of paper) version of the MDHAQ (**Fig. 1**) designed for the patient's initial visit (or, if introducing a database, initial visit for entry into a database) has been used by the senior author for more than two decades. The four-page version includes identical queries to the two-page version on the first two pages. The two additional pages list elements of a standard medical history: previous illnesses, surgeries, hospitalizations, family history, current medications, allergies, and

19. Please write below all pills that you took over the last TWO WEEKS, with or without a prescription. Include aspirin, birth control pills, pain pills, alternative therapy, health supplements, pills sold in health food stores:

NAME OF DRUG, MEDICINE OR ALTERNATIVE THERAPY	DOSE (if known)	How Many per day or week?	NAME OF DRUG, MEDICINE OR ALTERNATIVE THERAPY	DOSE (if known)	How Many Per day or week?
1.			7.		
2.			8.		
3.			9.		
4.			10.		
5.			11.		
6.			12.		

20. What is your current occupation? (If you are not working now, what was your past occupation?)

_____

21. At this time, are you?[Please check(✓)all that apply.]
__Working full time   __Retired
__Working part time   __Student
__Homemaker-full time __Disabled
__Seeking work   __Other (describe)_____

22. How many other people live at home with you? ____
[Please check (✓) who lives with you.]
__Spouse/partner   __Parents   __Sons or daughters
__I live alone   __Others (describe)_____

23. How many years of school have you completed?
Please circle the number of years of school:
1   2   3   4   5   6   7   8   9   10
11 12 13 14 15 16 17 18 19 20

24. Please write your weight: ____lbs. height: ___in.

Your Name_____ Today's Date_____ Time of Day_____ AM/PM
          First   Middle   Last

Street Address_____ City_____ State____ Zip_____

Telephone (___) _____ Social Security #_____ Date of Birth _____
          Area Code   Number   For Identification Purposes Only

SEX: ☐ Female   ETHNIC☐ Asian ☐ Hispanic ☐ Other   MARITAL STATUS: ☐ Single   ☐ Married ☐ Divorced
     ☐ Male   GROUP:☐ Black ☐ White   ☐ Widowed ☐ Separated

Please check if this questionnaire is completed ☐ entirely by patient OR ☐ with help from (name)_____

WE ASK YOU FOR CONSENT TO REVIEW YOUR RECORDS FOR MEDICAL RESEARCH AND TO CONTACT YOU IN THE FUTURE. YOUR CARE WILL NOT BE AFFECTED IF YOU ANSWER "NO."
I agree to allow information from my medical record to be reviewed for medical research, and for you to send me similar questionnaires in the future, which I am not required to answer. I understand that this information will remain confidential with my doctor and his or her research associates only. Please check (✓) in one box. Thank you!

   ☐ YES   ☐ NO   Signature_____ Date _____

I understand and agree that my doctor may share this information with colleagues at other medical research centers, in order to learn more about best treatments for my condition. Please check (✓) in one box. Thank you!

   ☐ YES   ☐ NO   Signature_____ Date _____

Please list the name, address, and telephone number of your primary care physician:
Name_____ Address_____
City, State ZIP _____ Telephone _____

Please list the name of your rheumatologist and insurance center:
Rheumatologist_____ Insurance_____

Please list the name, address, and telephone number of someone who lives at a different address from you, and who will be likely to know your whereabouts if we are unable to reach you:
Name_____ Address_____
City, State ZIP _____ Telephone_____ Relationship _____

Page 4 of 4   Thank you for completing this questionnaire to help keep track of your medical care.   R811NP4

FOR OFFICE USE ONLY: I have reviewed the questionnaire responses.
Date: _____   Signature_____

Copyright: Health Report Services, Telephone 615-470-5303, E-mail tedpincus@gmail.com

Fig. 1. (continued)

demographic data. This version also includes a request for patient consent in the initial consent and Health Insurance Portability and Accountability Act (HIPAA) forms, for review of medical records, future contact to analyze outcomes if the patient does not return to the same clinical setting, and for sharing the patient's data with other research colleagues for collaborative studies, while maintaining strict confidentiality.

STEP 2: ENTER PATIENT HISTORY INTO THE DATABASE

The patient history from the four-page MDHAQ is entered into the Access database. This may seem cumbersome and expensive. Entry into a database, however, whether by a physician or a transcriptionist if the data are dictated, involves no more effort than

Medical History Synopsis - Sample Patient #10003

| MR# SMP#10003 | Ph# : (555) 555-1212 | DOB: 07/04/1776 | Date Last Reviewed: 2006 |
| PCP : John H. Smith, M.D. | Ph# : (917) 555-1212 | Fax : (917) 555-1212 | |

Illnesses	Year (Age)	Illnesses	Year (Age)
Gastroesophogeal Reflux	2002 (69)	Dry Eyes	2002 (69)
Bronchitis	1999 (66)	Mental Illness	1996 (63)
Depression	1996 (63)	Heart Attack	1992 (59)
Stomach Ulcer	1986 (53)	Rheumatoid Arthritis	1974 (41)
Back or Spine Problems	1960 (27)	Severe Allergies	1943 (10)

Operations	Date	Location
Angioplasty	1992	St. Thomas Hospital, Nashville, TN
Deviated Septum	1980	Memorial Hospital- Chattanooga, Chattanooga, TN
Hemorrhoid	1978	Westside Medical Center, Nashville, TN
Hemorrhoid	1966	Memorial Hospital- Chattanooga, Chattanooga, TN
Deviated Septum	1951	Hackney's Clinic, Chattanooga, TN
Tonsillectomy	1938	Decherd Tennessee Clinic, Winchester, TN

Other Hospital Admissions	Date	Location
No Reported Hospitalizations		Nashville, TN

Drug Allergies
Motrin	Penicillin	Miacalcin Iu/Spray

Other Allergies
Molds	Pollens	Dust Mites	Grasses

Family History	Status (Age)	Illnesses / Cause of Death
Father	Dead (80)	Stroke
Mother	Dead (75)	Heart Attack
Brother 1	Dead (49)	Heart Attack

Social History
Marital Status: Married   **Education:** 16

Occupation: Real Estate   **Work Status:** Part-Time

Review of Systems
General:	Negative.
Skin:	Negative.
HEENT:	Positive for dry eyes, stuffy nose, dry mouth, smell or taste problems. Otherwise negative.
Respiratory	Positive for cough. Otherwise negative.
Cardiac:	Negative.
Genitourinary	Positive for heartburn, constipation. Otherwise negative.
GI:	Negative.
Neurologic:	Negative.
Musculoskeleta	Positive for muscle pain, muscle weakness, joint pain, back pain, neck pain. Otherwise negative.
Psychiatric	Positive for memory problems, sleeping problems. Otherwise negative.
Habits:	Negative.

Copyright © 2009: Health Report Services, Inc., Telephone: 646-460-4433, E-mail: tedpincus@gmail.com

Fig. 2. A report in standard format for the physician, generated from the patient history database. (*Courtesy of* Health Report Services, Copyright © 2009 Health Reports Service, Inc. Email: tedpincus@gmail.com.)

the current practice of typing the information into a paper or electronic medical record (EMR). Although information can be entered into a database as easily as into a medical narrative, the database presents a major advantage in capacities for updating and correcting, and for analyses in clinical research.

STEP 3: REPORT OF THE PATIENT HISTORY IN A STANDARD FORMAT FOR A PHYSICIAN

A report in the standard format for a patient history in a medical record is generated by the database (**Fig. 2**). Information in the report requires no additional typing or

PATIENT INFORMATION REVIEW - Sample Patient #10003

Our commitment to excellent medical care includes maintaining an accurate record of your major health information. We ask your help to assure that the record is correct and up to date by reviewing it at this time. Please make any additions on the right side or the back of this page. If there are no corrections, please mark where indicated to acknowledge you have reviewed this information.

Basic Information   Date of Last Update: 2006

☐ If all correct, please check; If not, please note changes below

Patient: Sample Patient #10003

Address 123 Anywhere Street
Springfield, USA 00911-0911

Phone: (555) 555-1212

SSN: SSN-11-2222

Demographic Information

☐ If all correct, please check; If not, please note changes below

Sex: Male   **Date Of Birth:** 7/4/1776

Education (years) 16

Occupation REAL ESTATE

Work Status Part-Time

Marital Status: Married

Contact Person Someone at a different address in case we cannot find you but need to tell you something such as abnormal lab test

☐ If all correct, please check; If not, please note changes below

Name: Emergency Contact Name

Address 789 Anywhere Road
Springfield, USA 00911-0911

Phone: (555) 555-6789

Relation Daughter

Primary Care Physician

☐ If all correct, please check; If not, please note changes below

Name: John H. Smith, MD

Address 911 Medical Center Drive
Springfield, USA 00911-0911

Phone: (917) 555-1212   **Fax:** (917) 555-1212

Copyright © 2009: Health Report Services, Inc., Telephone: 646-460-4433, E-mail: tedpincus@gmail.com

Fig. 3. A report for presentation to the patient at the next visit, generated from the patient history database. Patient history information from the database is listed on the left side of the page, with space on the right side for the patient to check if correct or to amend information that is incorrect. (*Courtesy of* Health Report Services, Copyright © 2009 Health Reports Service, Inc. Email: tedpincus@gmail.com.)

dictation, once entered into the database by a physician, assistant, data entry clerk, or anyone. Such a report has been generated by the Microsoft Access program on every patient seen by the senior author since 2000.

The physician's medical record note adds three components to the report provided by the patient: a chief complaint and present illness narrative (generally only two or three sentences); physical examination; and management plan. These components

PATIENT INFORMATION REVIEW - Sample Patient #10003

MEDICAL CONDITIONS	Year of Onset	☐ If all correct, please check; If not, please note changes below
Severe Allergies	YEAR	
Back or Spine Problems	YEAR	
Rheumatoid Arthritis	YEAR	
Stomach Ulcer	YEAR	
Heart Attack	YEAR	
Depression	YEAR	
Mental Illness	YEAR	
Bronchitis	YEAR	
Dry Eyes	YEAR	
Gastroesophogeal Reflux	YEAR	

SURGERIES	Year	Hospital (City/State)	☐ If all correct, please check; If not, please note changes below
Tonsillectomy	YEAR	General Hospital, Somewhere USA	
Deviated Septum	YEAR	General Hospital, Somewhere USA	
Hemorrhoid	YEAR	General Hospital, Somewhere USA	
Hemorrhoid	YEAR	General Hospital, Somewhere USA	
Deviated Septum	YEAR	General Hospital, Somewhere USA	
Angioplasty	YEAR	General Hospital, Somewhere USA	

HOSPITIALIZATIONS	Year	Hospital (City/State)	☐ If all correct, please check; If not, please note changes below
No Reported Hospitalizations	YEAR	General Hospital, Somewhere USA	

FAMILY MEDICAL HISTORY					☐ If all correct, please check; If not, please note changes below
Family Member	Alive or Deceased	Date of Birth	Year of Death	Major Health Conditions	
Father	Deceased	DOB	DOD	Stroke	
Mother	Deceased	DOB	DOD	Heart Attack	
Brother 1	Deceased	DOB	DOD	Heart Attack	

MEDICATION ALLERGIES	☐ If all correct, please check; If not, please note changes below
Miacalcin Iu/Spray	
Motrin	
Penicillin	

OTHER ALLERGIES	☐ If all correct, please check; If not, please note changes below
Dust Mites	
Grasses	
Molds	
Pollens	

Copyright © 2009: Health Report Services, Inc., Telephone: 646-460-4433, E-mail: tedpincus@gmail.com

Fig. 3. (*continued*)

can be entered through dictation and transcription, typing into an EMR, or other mechanism. The physical examination may also be in a format for entry into a database, through templates or standard entry screens. Most of the medical record note is provided by patient data entered into a database, rather than entered by the physician into a narrative medical note.

STEP 4: REPORT OF THE PATIENT HISTORY FOR REVIEW BY THE PATIENT

A second report is generated from the database (that also generated the physician report) for presentation to the patient, generally at the next visit (**Fig. 3**). The patient report may be presented in a computer or paper version. Patient history information

PT: Sample Patient #10003   **MR#:**   SMP#10003

Our records indicate that your last visit you were taking the medications listed below. Please review each medication and indicate whether you have taken or not over the last week. If you have taken the medication, please indicate how helpful the medication is and if you have any side effects from the medication.

			Number of Tabs Taken?	How Often?	Taken at this Dose?	Taken-Other Dose?	Stopped	If taken, how helpful is it? A lot Some None Not Sure No	Any side effects? Yes (Please Note)
Refill	Medication Name	Dosage							
☐	Aspirin	81mg	1	Once Daily	☐ _____	☐		__ __ __ __ __	_____
☐	Folic Acid	1mg	1	Once Daily	☐ _____	☐		__ __ __ __ __	_____
☐	methotrexate	2.5mg	5	Every Week	☐ _____	☐		__ __ __ __ __	_____
☐	prednisone	1mg	3	Once Daily	☐ _____	☐		__ __ __ __ __	_____
☐	Multivitamin Tablets	1tab	1	Once Daily	☐ _____	☐		__ __ __ __ __	_____
☐	Prevacid	30mg	1	Once Daily	☐ _____	☐		__ __ __ __ __	_____
☐	Procardia Xl	30mg	1	Once Daily	☐ _____	☐		__ __ __ __ __	_____
☐	Tums	500mg	1	As Needed	☐ _____	☐		__ __ __ __ __	_____
☐	Tylenol	500mg	1	As Needed	☐ _____	☐		__ __ __ __ __	_____
☐	Zocor	20mg	1	Once Daily	☐ _____	☐		__ __ __ __ __	_____

Please List Any New Medication

_____ _____ _____	☐ _____	☐	__ __ __ __ __
_____ _____ _____	☐ _____	☐	__ __ __ __ __
_____ _____ _____	☐ _____	☐	__ __ __ __ __
_____ _____ _____	☐ _____	☐	__ __ __ __ __
_____ _____ _____	☐ _____	☐	__ __ __ __ __

FOR OFFICE USE ONLY

DRUG CHANGES SINCE LAST VISIT (circle one):   NO   YES --   List all changes below

NEW DRUGS AND DOSAGE	CHANGE IN DOSAGE	DISCONTINUATION (BASIS)	D/C CODES
			NO efficacy TOXicity LOSS of efficacy MD orders PT refused ADMinistrative

Copyright © 2009: Health Report Services, Inc., Telephone: 646-460-4433, E-mail: tedpincus@gmail.com

Fig. 3. (*continued*)

from the database is listed on the left side of the page, with space on the right side for the patient to check if correct or to amend information that is incorrect.

A report used by the senior author since 2000 involves three pages in a pencil-and-paper format: page 1 lists demographic data, physician, insurance, and other information; page 2 lists past medical history including illnesses, surgeries, hospitalizations, and allergies; and page 3 lists medications recorded at the previous visit. The patient is invited to check if correct or make any changes. Pages 4 and 5 in this format are the two pages of the standard MDHAQ (similar to **Fig. 1**).

STEP 5: ENTRY OF CORRECTIONS INTO THE DATABASE

The final step is to enter corrections into the database so a more accurate history than initially recorded is available and propagated. This form of quality control requires no more time than typing the usual medical note into the Access software system. The Microsoft Access database used by the authors could be reprogrammed to an available EMR. In the future (at present in a few sites), a patient and physician might enter information directly into a database.

Availability of a database also facilitates analyses of research questions (eg, how many patients in a particular practice were taking methotrexate or a specific biologic agent, how many people being treated for rheumatoid arthritis had a history of pneumonia or joint replacement surgery). A database in the infrastructure of all rheumatology care obviates a need for specific registries and greatly reduces costs of assessing outcomes in patients with rheumatic diseases. Readers and EMR developers are invited to inquire about use of this system by contacting the senior author at tedpincus@gmail.com.

Criterion Contamination of Depression Scales in Patients with Rheumatoid Arthritis: The Need for Interpretation of Patient Questionnaires (as All Clinical Measures) in the Context of All Information About the Patient

Theodore Pincus, MD[a],*, Afton L. Hassett, PsyD[b],
Leigh F. Callahan, PhD[c]

KEYWORDS

- Minnesota multiphasic personality inventory (MMPI)
- Beck depression inventory (BDI)
- Centers for epidemiologic studies depression scale (CES-D)
- Criterion contamination

Development of questionnaires for completion by patients requires documentation of validity (ie, that the questionnaire measures what is thought to be measured) and reliability (ie, that a questionnaire measures the construct of interest consistently). These criteria are appropriate and required to interpret patient self-report information

Supported in part by research grants from the Arthritis Foundation and the Jack C. Massey Foundation.

[a] Division of Rheumatology, Department of Medicine, NYU Hospital for Joint Diseases, New York University School of Medicine, 301 East 17th Street, Room 1608, New York, NY 10003, USA
[b] Division of Rheumatology and Connective Tissue Research, Department of Medicine, UMDNJ-Robert Wood Johnson Medical School, New Brunswick, NJ
[c] School of Medicine and Gillings School of Global Public Health, University of North Carolina at Chapel Hill, Chapel Hill, NC, USA
* Corresponding author.
E-mail address: tedpincus@gmail.com (T. Pincus).

Rheum Dis Clin N Am 35 (2009) 861–864
doi:10.1016/j.rdc.2009.10.015
0889-857X/09/$ – see front matter © 2009 Elsevier Inc. All rights reserved.

correctly. At the same time, "validity" of information provided by a person may not necessarily be generalizable to all situations, and may depend on the context in which a patient provides the information.

A notable example of a need to consider context in interpreting patient self-report data can be seen in observations made in patients with rheumatoid arthritis (RA) based on their responses on questionnaires designed to identify depression and other psychological tendencies in the general population. For example, the Minnesota Multiphasic Personality Inventory (MMPI) consists of 566 statements to which the patient responds "true" or "false" that comprise 3 validity scales and 10 clinical scales.[1,2] Responses on 3 of the MMPI clinical scales have been validated to recognize trends to hypochondriasis, depression, and hysteria in subjects from the general population. Several reports indicated elevated scores in patients with RA on these 3 scales, some of which were interpreted as indicating that these patients had evidence of hypochondriasis, depression, and hysteria,[3–6] although disagreement has existed regarding interpretation of these findings.[7–10]

To better understand the implications of elevated scores on the MMPI Hypochondriasis, Depression, and Hysteria scales, analyses of responses of 34 individual RA patients from Wichita, Kansas, were compared to 130 age-matched control subjects and 23 area-matched control subjects.[11] As in all previous reports, elevated scores were seen in RA patients on the Hypochondriasis, Depression, and Hysteria scales. However, these elevations were found to result in large part from responses of "false" to such MMPI statements as "I am in just as good physical health as most of my friends" and "During the past few years I have been well most of the time," which are found on all three scales (**Box 1**).

The validity of the MMPI Hypochondriasis, Depression, and Hysteria scales was established in individuals who did not have any somatic disease. In these people, responses of "false" concerning good health differentiated subjects with tendencies to hypochondriasis, depression, and hysteria from normal subjects. At the same time, higher scores of patients with RA on these scales reflects evidence of disease, independent of possible psychological tendencies. The findings in RA patients agreed with predictions of 18 rheumatologists concerning which of the 117 statements that comprise the three MMPI Hypochondriasis, Depression, and Hysteria scales would be answered differently by RA patients, because of RA, than by subjects without chronic disease, without regard to psychological status. This phenomenon has been termed *criterion contamination*.[12]

Criterion contamination also has been recognized in responses of people with RA on depression scales,[12–14] including the original Beck Depression Inventory (BDI)[15] and the Centers for Epidemiologic Studies Depression Scale (CES-D).[16,17] Again, as with the MMPI, the validity of these questionnaires to identify individuals affected by depression had been established in young people, often graduate students, who did not have somatic disease and in whom somatic symptoms were characteristic of depression. However, items on the original BDI, such as "I can work about as well as before" or "I am no more worried about my health than usual," or on the CES-D, such as "I felt like everything I did was an effort" or "I could not get going" (see **Box 1**) would be interpreted as indicative of depression in a young person without somatic disease, but would be an accurate report of the status of an individual with RA. A revised version of the BDI, the Beck Depression Inventory-II (BDI-II), published in 1996, eliminated two of these six "somatic" items, to be less sensitive to somatic issues.[18,19]

The observations of criterion contamination in the original BDI and the CES-D, as well as the MMPI Hypochondriasis, Depression, and Hysteria scales, indicate that

---

Box 1
"Disease-related" individual items identified on widely used depression scales

MMPI[1,2]

   9. I am about as able to work as I ever was.[a]

  51. I am in just as good physical health as most of my friends.[a]

153. During the past few years I have been well most of the time.[a]

163. I do not tire quickly.[b]

243. I have few or no pains.[b]

Beck Depression Inventory[15]

15. I can work about as well as before.

16. I can sleep as well as usual.

17. I don't get more tired than usual.

18. My appetite is no worse than usual.

20. I am no more worried about my health than usual.

21. I have not noticed any recent change in my interest in sex.

Center for Epidemiologic Studies Depression Scale[16,17]

  2. I did not feel like eating; my appetite was poor.

  7. I felt that everything I did was an effort.

11. My sleep was restless.

20. I could not "get going."

[a] Found on each of three hypochondriasis, depression and hysteria scales.
[b] Found on each of two scales for hypochondriasis and hysteria scales.
From Pincus T, Callahan LF, Bradley LA, et al. Elevated MMPI scores for hypochondriasis, depression, and hysteria in patients with rheumatoid arthritis reflect disease rather than psychological status. Arthritis Rheum 1986;29:1456–66.

---

patient questionnaire measures must be examined in light of all information about a person, particularly a medical diagnosis, to interpret their significance. "Validity" of a questionnaire may not necessarily be generalizable to all populations. The population in which a questionnaire has been validated may differ from a study population, and caution must be exercised in interpreting the data.

REFERENCES

1. McKinley JC, Hathaway SR. The identification and measurement of the psycho-neuroses in medical practice: the Minnesota Multiphasic Personality Inventory. JAMA 1943;122:161–7.
2. Colligan RC, Osborne D, Swenson WM, et al. The MMPI, a contemporary normative study. New York: Praeger Scientific; 1983.
3. Moos RH, Solomon GF. Minnesota Multiphasic Personality Inventory response patterns in patients with rheumatoid arthritis. J Psychosom Res 1964;8:17–28.
4. Nalven FB, O'Brien JF. Personality patterns of rheumatoid arthritic patients. Arthritis Rheum 1964;7:18–28.
5. Polley HF, Swenson WM, Steinhilber RM. Personality characteristics of patients with rheumatoid arthritis. Psychosomatics 1970;11:45–9.

6. Spergel P, Ehrlich GE, Glass D. The rheumatoid arthritic personality: a psycho-diagnostic myth. Psychosomatics 1978;19:79–86.

7. Liang MH, Rogers M, Larson M, et al. The psychosocial impact of systemic lupus erythematosus and rheumatoid arthritis. Arthritis Rheum 1984;27:13–9.

8. Wolfe F, Cathey MA, Kleinheksel SM, et al. Psychological status in primary fibrositis and fibrositis associated with rheumatoid arthritis. J Rheumatol 1984;11:500–6.

9. Smythe HA. Problems with the MMPI [editorial]. J Rheumatol 1984;11:417–8.

10. Colligan RC, Osborne D, Swenson WM, et al. The aging MMPI: development of contemporary norms. Mayo Clin Proc 1984;59:377–90.

11. Pincus T, Callahan LF, Bradley LA, et al. Elevated MMPI scores for hypochondriasis, depression, and hysteria in patients with rheumatoid arthritis reflect disease rather than psychological status. Arthritis Rheum 1986;29:1456–66.

12. Callahan LF, Kaplan MR, Pincus T. The Beck Depression Inventory, Center for Epidemiological Studies Depression Scale (CES-D), and General Well-being Schedule depression subscale in rheumatoid arthritis: criterion contamination of responses. Arthritis Care Res 1991;4:3–11.

13. Blalock SJ, DeVellis RF, Brown GK, et al. Validity of the Center for Epidemiological Studies Depression Scale in arthritis populations. Arthritis Rheum 1989;32:991–7.

14. Pincus T, Callahan LF. Depression scales in rheumatoid arthritis: criterion contamination in interpretation of patient responses. Patient Educ Couns 1993;20:133–43.

15. Beck AT, Ward CH, Mendelson M, et al. An inventory for measuring depression. Arch Gen Psychiatry 1961;4:561–71.

16. Radloff LS. The CES-D scale: a self-report depression scale for research in the general population. Appl Psychol Meas 1977;1:385–401.

17. Radloff LS, Teri L. Use of the Center for Epidemiological Studies-Depression Scale with older adults. In: Brink TL, editor. Clinical gerontology: a guide to assessment and intervention. New York: Haworth Press; 1986. p. 119–35.

18. Beck AT, Steer RA, Brown GK. Manual for the beck depression inventory-II. San Antonio (TX): Psychological Corporation; 1996.

19. Beck AT, Steer RA, Ball R, et al. Comparison of Beck depression inventories-IA and -II in psychiatric outpatients. J Pers Assess 1996;67:588–97.

Clues on the MDHAQ to Identify Patients with Fibromyalgia and Similar Chronic Pain Conditions

Theodore Pincus, MD[a],*, Afton L. Hassett, PsyD[b],
Leigh F. Callahan, PhD[c]

KEYWORDS

- Fibromyalgia/chronic pain conditions • Pain
- MDHAQ • Fatigue

Patients with fibromyalgia and similar chronic pain conditions are among the most complex for physicians. Because they may report many different types of symptoms, they often have extensive and expensive evaluations that generally do not provide a diagnosis. These patients often are seen by several doctors, with an approach that many possible diagnoses must be "ruled out" through elaborate testing. In some cases, a diagnosis of fibromyalgia/chronic pain conditions is apparent clinically, although it is a source of discomfort to doctors and patients to have a negative test rather than a pattern that might point to a recognizable disease entity.

Patients with fibromyalgia/chronic pain conditions typically report high levels of pain and fatigue, and multiple symptoms on a review of systems. These phenomena generally are reflected in high scores on visual analog scales (VAS) or pain, fatigue, and patient global estimate on questionnaires, such as the health assessment questionnaire (HAQ) and multidimensional HAQ (MDHAQ) (see "The HAQ Compared with the MDHAQ: "Keep It Simple, Stupid" (KISS), with Feasibility and Clinical Value as Primary Criteria for Patient Questionnaires in Usual Clinical Care," by Pincus and

Supported in part by research grants from the Arthritis Foundation and the Jack C. Massey Foundation.

[a] Division of Rheumatology, Department of Medicine, New York University School of Medicine, New York, NY 10003, USA

[b] Division of Rheumatology and Connective Tissue Research, Department of Medicine, UMDNJ-Robert Wood Johnson Medical School, New Brunswick, NJ

[c] School of Medicine and Gillings School of Global Public Health, University of North Carolina at Chapel Hill, Chapel Hill, NC, USA

* Corresponding author. Division of Rheumatology, Department of Medicine, NYU School of Medicine, New York, NY 10003, USA

E-mail address: tedpincus@gmail.com (T. Pincus).

Rheum Dis Clin N Am 35 (2009) 865–869
doi:10.1016/j.rdc.2009.10.013
0889-857X/09/$ – see front matter © 2009 Elsevier Inc. All rights reserved.

Swearingen, in this issue).[1,2] VAS scores usually are greater than 6; therefore, routine assessment of patient index data 3 (RAPID3) composite scores of physical function, pain, and patient global estimate, all scored 0 to 10, are greater than 12, suggestive of high severity in patients with rheumatoid arthritis (RA) (see "RAPID3, an Index to Assess and Monitor Patients with Rheumatoid Arthritis, Without Formal Joint Counts: Similar Results to DAS28 and CDAI in Clinical Trials and Clinical Care," by Pincus T, Yazici Y, Bergman MJ, in this issue).[3,4]

Some health professionals have suggested that results of a HAQ or MDHAQ are "valid" only in RA and other inflammatory rheumatic diseases, as patients with fibromyalgia may have pain scores as high as—and generally higher than—patients with RA. A poster was presented at a major rheumatology meeting, entitled "Fake"—suggesting that individuals reporting high pain scores without evidence of inflammatory disease might be regarded as not giving valid information. This view denigrates the patients and ignores recent observations concerning the neuroscience of pain in patients with fibromyalgia/chronic pain conditions.[5]

Another approach to understanding information on patient questionnaires that may appear invalid or incorrect initially might be to attempt to recognize patterns on a questionnaire that might provide informative clues to the presence of fibromyalgia/chronic pain conditions. Patterns on the MDHAQ observed in usual clinical care provide capacity to recognize patients with fibromyalgia/chronic pain conditions. Two reports summarized in this article might provide a cost-effective approach to identify such patients.

It was recognized in 1990[6] that patients with fibromyalgia/chronic pain conditions have high scores on a pain VAS but often had low scores on the physical function scale on a modified health assessment questionnaire (MHAQ),[7] which led to a MDHAQ.[8,9] A ratio of pain (scored 0–10 on a VAS) to physical function (scored 1–4 on an MHAQ in use during the 1980s) of 5 or more was seen in approximately one-half of the patients with fibromyalgia but in no patients with RA (**Fig. 1**).[6] As with all quantitative measures in rheumatology, including laboratory tests, some fibromyalgia patients had a low ratio in the normal range.[6]

These results were extended to analyses using the MDHAQ,[8,9] which includes a fatigue VAS and a symptom checklist for review of systems (see "The HAQ Compared with the MDHAQ: "Keep It Simple, Stupid" (KISS), with Feasibility and Clinical Value as Primary Criteria for Patient Questionnaires in Usual Clinical Care," by Pincus and Swearingen, in this issue) (**Fig. 2**). A ratio of pain VAS score to physical function score was again elevated in patients with fibromyalgia/chronic pain conditions.[10] Furthermore, a ratio of a fatigue VAS score to physical function score was also elevated, at even higher levels (see **Fig. 2**).[10] In addition, patients who reported more than 20 symptoms on a checklist of 60 symptoms in review of systems were substantially more likely to have a fibromyalgia/chronic pain disorder than an inflammatory rheumatic disease.[10] The questionnaire scores differed between the two patient groups at levels similar to difference in the erythrocyte sedimentation rate (ESR).

As is the case with all medical tests, data from a patient questionnaire must be interpreted in light of medical history, physical examination, laboratory tests, and imaging studies. In patients with RA, scores for RAPID3 on the MDHAQ provide useful classification of high (>12 on a 0–30 scale), moderate (6.1–12.0), and low severity (3.1–6.0) and remission (≤3).[4] In patients with fibromyalgia/chronic pain conditions, RAPID3 scores generally indicate high severity, based on frequent scores for pain and global estimate greater than 6, for a total RAPID3 score of at least 12. Health professionals must examine the pattern, however, and all other information about patients, to interpret questionnaire data accurately. The information is particularly helpful in patients who may meet criteria for inflammatory

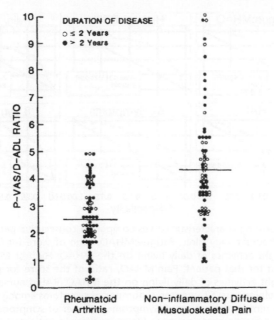

Fig. 1. Ratio of scores on a pain VAS (P-VAS) to scale scores of difficulty in performance of eight activities of daily living (D-ADL) in 75 RA patients and 75 patients with noninflammatory diffuse musculoskeletal pain. Bars show the mean ratio for each group. (*From* Callahan LF, Pincus T. The P-VAS/D-ADL ratio: a clue from a self-report questionnaire to distinguish rheumatoid arthritis from noninflammatory diffuse musculoskeletal pain. Arthritis Rheum 1990;33:1317–22; with permission.)

disease, such as RA or systemic lupus erythematosus (SLE), but also may have extensive symptomatology based on fibromyalgia/chronic pain conditions, which may apply to as many as 20% to 30% of patients with inflammatory diseases.[11,12]

All rheumatology laboratory tests are characterized by false-positive and false-negative results (see "Laboratory Tests to Assess Patients with Rheumatoid Arthritis: Advantages and Limitations," by Pincus and Sokka, in this issue). For example, the ESR or C-reactive protein may be as high or higher in patients with tuberculosis or lymphoma compared to many patients with RA. This phenomenon does not render the ESR or C-reactive protein "invalid" in patients with RA, but again indicates that results of any medical tests require interpretation by a knowledgeable physician. Similarly, a patient questionnaire measure or ratio of scores, interpreted correctly, with complementary data from patient history, physical examination, laboratory tests, and imaging studies, can help guide diagnosis and management with appropriate interpretation.

According to a biomedical model,[13] the traditional paradigm of twentieth century medicine, a reductionist perspective seeks to identify a single cause or single cure for a given disease. Thus, in a simple interpretation of "content validity," a patient who checks headache, shortness of breath, or abdominal discomfort on a MDHAQ symptom checklist should receive an evaluation for each of these symptoms. Patients who check all three symptoms at a given time, however, while sitting in a waiting room in an outpatient department, are unlikely to have substantial somatic problems with any of the three systems in most situations, particularly if they report no functional disability. The MDHAQ allows quantitation of a "positive review of systems" through a standard checklist—a standard format converts descriptive

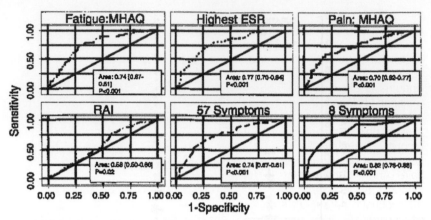

Fig. 2. Receiver operating characteristic curves comparing consecutive patients with RA or fibromyalgia in a rheumatology clinic. Fatigue:MHAQ, ratio of score for fatigue on a VAS to the score for eight activities of daily living on the MHAQ; Highest ESR, highest value of the ESR recorded for that patient; Pain:MHAQ, ratio of the score for pain on the VAS to the score for eight activities of daily living on the MHAQ; RAI, rheumatology attitudes index to measure helplessness; 57 Symptoms, number of symptoms among 57 symptoms reported as being present by the patient; 8 Symptoms, number of symptoms among 8 of 57 symptoms, identified by rheumatologists as likely to differ in patients with fibromyalgia, compared with those with RA. (*From* DeWalt DA, Reed GW, Pincus T. Further clues to recognition of patients with fibromyalgia from a simple 2-page patient multidimensional health assessment questionnaire (MDHAQ). Clin Exp Rheumatol 2004;22:453–61.)

information into quantitative scientific information (see "Patient Questionnaires in Rheumatoid Arthritis: Advantages and Limitations as a Quantitative, Standardized Scientific Medical History," by Pincus T, et al, in this issue).

Perhaps a most important lesson from these observations should be reiterated: all medical data—laboratory tests, imaging procedures, and questionnaire responses—require interpretation by a treating physician in formulation of management decisions. Data from the MDHAQ in patients with RA, fibromyalgia, or both offer important examples of this lesson. A patient may not need an extensive evaluation for a particular symptom, if it is reported in a pattern that indicates a high likelihood that a specific cause will not be identified.

REFERENCES

1. Callahan LF, Smith WJ, Pincus T. Self-report questionnaires in five rheumatic diseases: comparisons of health status constructs and associations with formal education level. Arthritis Care Res 1989;2:122–31.
2. Pincus T, Sokka T. Can a Multi-Dimensional Health Assessment Questionnaire (MDHAQ) and Routine Assessment of Patient Index Data (RAPID) scores be informative in patients with all rheumatic diseases? Best Pract Res Clin Rheumatol 2007;21:733–53.
3. Pincus T, Swearingen CJ, Bergman M, et al. RAPID3 (routine assessment of patient index data 3), a rheumatoid arthritis index without formal joint counts for routine care: proposed severity categories compared to DAS and CDAI categories. J Rheumatol 2008;35:2136–47.

4. Pincus T. Can RAPID3, an index without formal joint counts or laboratory tests, serve to guide rheumatologists in tight control of rheumatoid arthritis in usual clinical care? Bull NYU Hosp Jt Dis 2009;67:254–66.

5. Ablein K, Clauw DJ. From fibrositis to functional somatic syndromes to a bell-shaped curve of pain and sensory sensitivity: evolution of a clinical construct. Rheum Dis Clin N Am 2009;35:233–51.

6. Callahan LF, Pincus T. The P-VAS/D-ADL ratio: a clue from a self-report questionnaire to distinguish rheumatoid arthritis from non-inflammatory diffuse musculoskeletal pain. Arthritis Rheum 1990;33:1317–22.

7. Pincus T, Summey JA, Soraci SA Jr, et al. Assessment of patient satisfaction in activities of daily living using a modified Stanford health assessment questionnaire. Arthritis Rheum 1983;26:1346–53.

8. Pincus T, Swearingen C, Wolfe F. Toward a multidimensional health assessment questionnaire (MDHAQ): assessment of advanced activities of daily living and psychological status in the patient friendly health assessment questionnaire format. Arthritis Rheum 1999;42:2220–30.

9. Pincus T, Sokka T, Kautiainen H. Further development of a physical function scale on a multidimensional health assessment questionnaire for standard care of patients with rheumatic diseases. J Rheumatol 2005;32:1432–9.

10. DeWalt DA, Reed GW, Pincus T. Further clues to recognition of patients with fibromyalgia from a simple 2-page patient multidimensional health assessment questionnaire (MDHAQ). Clin Exp Rheumatol 2004;22:453–61.

11. Wolfe F, Cathey MA, Kleinheksel SM. Fibrositis (fibromyalgia) in rheumatoid arthritis. J Rheumatol 1984;11:814–8.

12. Wolfe F, Petri M, Alarcon GS, et al. Fibromyalgia, systemic lupus erythematosus (SLE), and evaluation of SLE activity. J Rheumatol 2009;36:82–8.

13. Engel GL. The need for a new medical model: a challenge for biomedicine. Science 1977;196:129–36.

Index

Note: Page numbers of article titles are in **boldface** type.

Rheum Dis Clin N Am 35 (2009) 871–875
doi:10.1016/S0889-857X(09)00109-4
0889-857X/09/$ – see front matter © 2009 Elsevier Inc. All rights reserved.

rheumatic.theclinics.com

United States Postal Service

Statement of Ownership, Management, and Circulation
(All Periodicals Publications Except Requestor Publications)

1. Publication Title	2. Publication Number	3. Filing Date
Rheumatic Disease Clinics of North America	0 0 6 - 2 7 2	9/15/09

4. Issue Frequency	5. Number of Issues Published Annually	6. Annual Subscription Price
Feb, May, Aug, Nov	4	$244.00

7. Complete Mailing Address of Known Office of Publication (Not printer) (Street, city, county, state, and ZIP+4®)

Elsevier Inc.
360 Park Avenue South
New York, NY 10010-1710

Contact Person: Stephen Bushing
Telephone (Include area code): 215-239-3688

8. Complete Mailing Address of Headquarters or General Business Office of Publisher (Not printer)

Elsevier Inc., 360 Park Avenue South, New York, NY 10010-1710

9. Full Names and Complete Mailing Addresses of Publisher, Editor, and Managing Editor (Do not leave blank)

Publisher (Name and complete mailing address)

John Schrefer, Elsevier, Inc., 1600 John F. Kennedy Blvd. Suite 1800, Philadelphia, PA 19103-2899

Editor (Name and complete mailing address)

Rachel Glover, Elsevier, Inc., 1600 John F. Kennedy Blvd. Suite 1800, Philadelphia, PA 19103-2899

Managing Editor (Name and complete mailing address)

Catherine Bewick, Elsevier, Inc., 1600 John F. Kennedy Blvd. Suite 1800, Philadelphia, PA 19103-2899

10. Owner (Do not leave blank. If the publication is owned by a corporation, give the name and address of the corporation immediately followed by the names and addresses of all stockholders owning or holding 1 percent or more of the total amount of stock. If not owned by a corporation, give the names and addresses of the individual owners. If owned by a partnership or other unincorporated firm, give its name and address as well as those of each individual owner. If the publication is published by a nonprofit organization, give its name and address.)

Full Name	Complete Mailing Address
Wholly owned subsidiary of	4520 East-West Highway
Reed/Elsevier, US holdings	Bethesda, MD 20814

11. Known Bondholders, Mortgagees, and Other Security Holders Owning or Holding 1 Percent or More of Total Amount of Bonds, Mortgages, or Other Securities. If none, check box ☐

Full Name	Complete Mailing Address
N/A	

12. Tax Status (For completion by nonprofit organizations authorized to mail at nonprofit rates) (Check one)
The purpose, function, and nonprofit status of this organization and the exempt status for federal income tax purposes:
☐ Has Not Changed During Preceding 12 Months
☐ Has Changed During Preceding 12 Months (Publisher must submit explanation of change with this statement)

PS Form 3526, September 2007 (Page 1 of 3 (Instructions Page 3)) PSN 7530-01-000-9931 PRIVACY NOTICE: See our Privacy policy in www.usps.com

---

13. Publication Title	14. Issue Date for Circulation Data Below
Rheumatic Disease Clinics of North America	May 2009

15. Extent and Nature of Circulation		Average No. Copies Each Issue During Preceding 12 Months	No. Copies of Single Issue Published Nearest to Filing Date
a. Total Number of Copies (Net press run)		1925	1800
b. Paid Circulation (By Mail and Outside the Mail)	(1) Mailed Outside-County Paid Subscriptions Stated on PS Form 3541. (Include paid distribution above nominal rate, advertiser's proof copies, and exchange copies)	749	667
	(2) Mailed In-County Paid Subscriptions Stated on PS Form 3541 (Include paid distribution above nominal rate, advertiser's proof copies, and exchange copies)		
	(3) Paid Distribution Outside the Mails Including Sales Through Dealers and Carriers, Street Vendors, Counter Sales, and Other Paid Distribution Outside USPS®	543	473
	(4) Paid Distribution by Other Classes Mailed Through the USPS (e.g. First-Class Mail®)		
c. Total Paid Distribution (Sum of 15b (1), (2), (3), and (4))		1292	1140
d. Free or Nominal Rate Distribution (By Mail and Outside the Mail)	(1) Free or Nominal Rate Outside-County Copies Included on PS Form 3541	64	87
	(2) Free or Nominal Rate In-County Copies Included on PS Form 3541		
	(3) Free or Nominal Rate Copies Mailed at Other Classes Through the USPS (e.g. First-Class Mail)		
	(4) Free or Nominal Rate Distribution Outside the Mail (Carriers or other means)		
e. Total Free or Nominal Rate Distribution (Sum of 15d (1), (2), (3) and (4))		64	87
f. Total Distribution (Sum of 15c and 15e)		1356	1227
g. Copies not Distributed (See instructions to publishers #4 (page 3))		569	573
h. Total (Sum of 15f and g)		1925	1800
i. Percent Paid (15c divided by 15f times 100)		95.28%	92.91%

16. Publication of Statement of Ownership
☐ If the publication is a general publication, publication of this statement is required. Will be printed in the November 2009 issue of this publication. ☐ Publication not required

17. Signature and Title of Editor, Publisher, Business Manager, or Owner

[signature] Stephen R. Bushing – Subscription Services Coordinator

Date: September 15, 2009

I certify that all information furnished on this form is true and complete. I understand that anyone who furnishes false or misleading information on this form or who omits material or information requested on the form may be subject to criminal sanctions (including fines and imprisonment) and/or civil sanctions (including civil penalties).

PS Form 3526, September 2007 (Page 2 of 3)

Moving?

Make sure your subscription moves with you!

To notify us of your new address, find your **Clinics Account Number** (located on your mailing label above your name), and contact customer service at:

Email: journalscustomerservice-usa@elsevier.com

800-654-2452 (subscribers in the U.S. & Canada)
314-447-8871 (subscribers outside of the U.S. & Canada)

Fax number: 314-447-8029

Elsevier Health Sciences Division
Subscription Customer Service
3251 Riverport Lane
Maryland Heights, MO 63043

*To ensure uninterrupted delivery of your subscription, please notify us at least 4 weeks in advance of move.

Printed and bound by CPI Group (UK) Ltd, Croydon, CR0 4YY

03/10/2024

01040462-0018